Practical
Gastrointestinal
Endoscopy
The Fundamentals

THIS BELONGS TO:

RUTHERFORD MORISSON

DO <u>NOT</u> REMOVE

D1494367

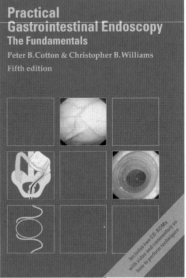

Practical Gastrointestinal Endoscopy
The Fundamentals

Peter B. Cotton
MD FRCP, FRCS
Director, Digestive Disease Center
Medical University of South Carolina
Charleston, South Carolina USA

Christopher B. Williams
MA, BM, BCh, FRCP
Endoscopy Unit
St Mark's Hospital for Colorectal and Intestinal Disorders
Harrow, London UK

FIFTH EDITION

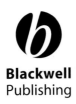

Blackwell
Publishing

First published 1980 by Blackwell Science Ltd
Reprinted 1981
Second edition 1982 by Blackwell Science Ltd
Reprinted 1984, 1985, 1987, 1988
Third edition 1990 by Blackwell Science Ltd
Reprinted 1991
Fourth edition 1996 by Blackwell Science Ltd
Reprinted 1997 (twice), 1999, 2000
Fifth edition 2003 by Blackwell Publishing Ltd
Reprinted 2003

Library of Congress Cataloging-in-Publication Data

Cotton, Peter B.
Practical gastrointestinal endoscopy: the fundamentals/Peter B. Cotton,
Christopher B. Williams–5th ed.
      p.; cm.
Includes bibliographical references and index.
ISBN 1-4051-0235-7
1 Gastroscopy.
[DNLM: 1 Gastrointestinal Diseases–diagnosis. 2 Endoscopy. WI
141 C851p 2003] I Williams, Christopher B. (Christopher Beverley) II Title.
RC804.G3 C68 2003
616.3'307545–dc21   2002151138

ISBN 1-4051-2118-1

A catalogue record for this title is available from the British Library

Set in 9/11½ pt Palatino by Sparks Computer Solutions Ltd, Oxford, UK
Printed and bound in Denmark by Narayana Press, Odder

Commissioning Editor: Alison Brown
Editorial Assistant: Elizabeth Callaghan
Production Editor: Jonathan Rowley
Production Controller: Chris Downs

For further information on Blackwell Publishing, visit our website:
www.blackwellpublishing.com

Contents

Preface to the fifth edition

Our earlier book, *Practical Gastrointestinal Endoscopy*, 4th edition (1996), was popular with a broad spectrum of endoscopists, from beginners to the most experienced. The field has become even more complex since that time, and it is increasingly difficult to cater to all needs in a single book. As a result, we have made several important conceptual changes. This book now focuses on the fundamentals of standard endoscopy practice, i.e. the core information which should be learned during the first year or so of training, and which remains the basis on which all of our endoscopic skills continue to build.

We have removed from the original text of *Practical Gastrointestinal Endoscopy* all of the advanced techniques (like ERCP), and also the content aimed mainly at managers and teachers. We then updated the remaining core sections, and complemented the text with two CD-Roms, concerning upper endoscopy, and colonoscopy, which should greatly enhance the educational experience. At the same time we are developing other resources concerning advanced endoscopy techniques, which we hope will be useful to senior trainees and practitioners. They will be published also by Blackwell Publishing, on-line and in print. By these means we intend to provide comprehensive resources for endoscopists at all levels of practice. We believe these plans are consistent with the changing learning and publishing environments, and hope that they meet our goal of enhancing the availability of high-quality endoscopic services to all patients who need them.

Peter B. Cotton
Christopher B. Williams
2003

Preface to the first edition

The human gut is long and tortuous. Diagnosis and localisation of its afflictions relied for many decades on barium radiology, which provides indirect data in black and white. Man is by nature inquisitive and direct inspection in colour is instinctively preferable and probably more accurate. Rigid open-ended instruments allow direct visual examination (and biopsy sampling) of only the proximal 40 cm and distal 25 cm of the gut. Semiflexible lens gastroscopes were introduced in the 1930s and 1940s and used by a few experts; examinations were uncomfortable and incomplete, and biopsy facilities were poor.

The situation has changed dramatically since the late 1960s with the introduction of fully flexible and manoeuvrable endoscopes. Upper gastrointestinal (GI) endoscopy is now a routine procedure which has superseded the barium meal as the primary diagnostic tool. Duodenoscopy allows direct cannulation of the papilla of Vater for cholangiography and pancreatography (ERCP). The whole colon can be examined, and methods are available for small intestinal endoscopy. Tissue specimens can be removed from all of these areas under direct vision, using biopsy forceps, cytology brushes and snare loops.

A further revolution occurred in the late 1970s with the arrival of endoscopic therapy. Transendoscopic snare removal has revolutionized the management of polyps, and flexible endoscopes now allow removal of foreign bodies, sphincterotomy for gallstones, insertion of stents, dilation of strictures, and direct attack on bleeding lesions and tumours.

GI endoscopy is a skill which requires motivation, determination and dexterity. Patients may suffer if examinations are not performed correctly, and endoscopic techniques themselves may fall into disrepute if results are suboptimal or unnecessary complications occur. The speed of development and the consequent clinical demand for endoscopy initially outstripped the evolution of training facilities. Many of the present 'experts' (including the authors) were self-taught, but instruction and experience of endoscopy should now be an integral part of GI training programmes.

This volume attempts to provide a basic framework for this process, and includes some 'tricks of the trade' which we find helpful.

Peter B. Cotton
Christopher B. Williams
1980

Acknowledgements

Peter Cotton gratefully acknowledges advice and help from several professional colleagues, especially Rob Hawes, Mike Wallace, Mark Delegge, Willie Webb, and Phyllis Malpas, and continuing expert secretarial assistance from Rita Oden, and the support of other staff of the Digestive Disease Center, Charleston, South Carolina.

Christopher Williams particularly acknowledges the support of Dr Christina Williams, and also that of his colleagues at St Mark's Hospital, London, especially Dr Brian Saunders. His colonoscopy CD-Rom carries its own credits, but owes much to the technical wizardry of Stephen Beston.

Note on the fifth edition

We have, on the advice of our publishers, adopted American spelling for this edition.

Apologies

For convenience, we continue to refer to doctors as 'he', and nurses as 'she', recognizing that these attributions are increasingly incorrect.

The Endoscopy Unit and Staff

Most endoscopists, and especially beginners, focus on the individual procedures and have little appreciation of the extensive infrastructure that is now necessary for efficient and safe activity. Aging experts can remember practicing with one instrument, a makeshift room and, maybe, a passing nurse. Now many of us work in large units with multiple procedure rooms full of complex electronic equipment, with space dedicated to preparation, recovery and reporting, in collaboration with teams of specially trained nurses and support staff. Endoscopy has become a sophisticated industry. More and more units resemble operating room suites—but with a human touch. Endoscopists are also learning (often painfully) some of the imperatives of surgical practice, such as efficient scheduling, disinfection and safe sedation/anesthesia. Setting up and running an endoscopy unit is a complex topic with an expanding literature, of particular interest to directors and nurse managers.

Endoscopy is a team activity, requiring the collaborative talents of many people of different backgrounds and training. It is difficult to overstate the importance of an appropriate environment and professional support staff, in order to maintain patient comfort and safety, and to optimize clinical outcomes. Procedures are performed by many different types of doctor, including gastroenterologists, surgeons, internists (general physicians), some family practitioners and radiologists. Nowadays some procedures are performed by specially trained nurses. There are also many different types of supporting staff.

STAFF

Specially trained endoscopy nurses are essential.

They have many important functions, including to:
- prepare patients for their procedures, physically and mentally;
- set up all of the necessary equipment;
- assist the endoscopist during procedures;
- monitor patients' safety, sedation and recovery;
- clean, disinfect and process equipment;
- maintain quality control.

Technicians and nursing aides may contribute to these functions. Large units need a variety of other staff, to handle reception, transport, reporting and equipment management.

FACILITIES

The modern endoscopy unit has areas designed for many different functions. Like a hotel or airport (or Victorian household),
the endoscopy unit should have a smart public face ('upstairs'),
and a more functional back hall ('downstairs'). From the patient's
perspective, endoscopy consists of areas devoted to reception,
preparation, procedure, recovery and discharge. Supporting
these activities are a series of other functions, which include
scheduling, cleaning, preparation, maintenance and storage of
equipment, reporting and archiving, and staff management.

Procedure rooms

These have certain key requirements. In general they should:
• not be cluttered or intimidating, because most patients are not
sedated when they enter. The room should resemble a modern
kitchen rather than an operating room.
• be large enough to allow a patient stretcher trolley to be rotated
on its axis, and to accommodate all of the equipment and staff
(and any emergency team), but also compact enough for efficient
function.
• be laid out with the specific functions in mind, keeping nursing and doctor spheres of activity separate (Fig. 1.1), and minimizing exposed trailing electrical cables and pipes.
Each room should have:
• piped oxygen and suction (two lines);
• lighting that is focused for nursing activities, but not dazzling
to the patient or endoscopist;

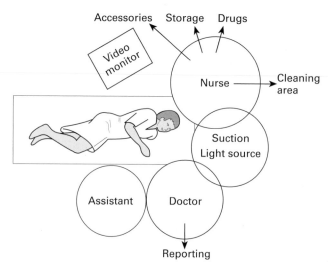

Fig. 1.1 Functional planning—spheres of activity.

- video monitors (for the endoscopy image and monitoring outputs) placed conveniently for the endoscopist and assistants;
- adequate counter space for accessories, and a large sink for dirty equipment;
- storage space for the equipment required on a daily basis;
- systems of communication with the charge nurse desk, and emergency call;
- disposal systems for hazardous materials.

Peri-procedure areas

The peri-procedure areas that patients encounter include:
- reception, and waiting for patients and accompanying persons.
- preparation (safety checking, consent, undressing, intravenous (IV) access).
- recovery. This should be separate from the preparation area—so that patients coming in are not mixed with those going out (for obvious reasons)—but adjacent for efficient nursing management.
- postprocedure interview and discharge. A private area must be available for sensitive consultations.

Staff areas

The endoscopy unit also has many support areas that patients do not see, including:
- a central focus workstation—this is needed in a unit of more than three endoscopy rooms; like the bridge of a ship, it is where the nurse captain of the day controls and steers the whole operation;
- endoscope storage, cleaning and disinfection;
- storage of all other equipment, including an emergency cart;
- medication storage;
- reporting;
- management office;
- staff belongings and refreshments.

MANAGEMENT AND BEHAVIOR

Such a complex organization requires efficient management and leadership. This works best as a collaborative exercise between the medical director of endoscopy, and the chief nurse or endoscopy nurse manager. They must be skilled in handling people (doctors, staff and patients), complex equipment and significant financial resources. They must develop and maintain good working relationships with many departments within the hospital (such as radiology, pathology, sterile processing, anesthesia, bioengineering), as well as numerous manufacturers and vendors. They need to be fully cognizant of all of the many local and national regulations which now impact on endoscopy practice.

The wise endoscopist will embrace the team approach, and realize that maintaining an atmosphere of collegiality and mutual respect is essential for efficiency, job satisfaction and staff retention, and for optimal patient outcomes. Sadly, patients sometimes tend to be packaged as mere commodities during the endoscopy process. Treating our customers (and those who accompany them) with respect and courtesy is fundamental. Always assume that patients are listening, even if apparently sedated, so never chatter about irrelevances in their presence. Never eat or drink in patient areas. Background music is appreciated by many patients and staff.

DOCUMENTATION

Information for patients (such as explanatory brochures and maps) is discussed in Chapter 3 (see 'Patient preparation').

The agreed policies of the unit (including regulations dictated by the hospital and national organizations) are enshrined in an Endoscopy Unit Procedure Manual (Fig. 1.2). This must be easily available, constantly updated, and frequently consulted.

Day-to-day documentation includes details of staff and room usage, disinfection processes, instrument and accessory use and problems, as well as the procedure reports.

Procedure reports

Usually, two reports are generated for each procedure—one by the nurses, and one by the endoscopist.

Nurse's report

The nurse's report usually takes the form of a preprinted 'flow sheet', with places to record all of the preprocedure safety checks, vital signs, use of sedation/analgesia and other medications, monitoring of vital signs and patient responses, equipment and accessory usage, and image documentation. It concludes with a copy of the discharge instructions given to the patient.

Endoscopist's report

The endoscopist's report includes the patient's demographics, reasons for the procedure (indications), specific medical risks and precautions, sedation/analgesia, findings, diagnostic specimens, treatments, conclusions, follow-up plans and any unplanned events (complications). Endoscopists use many re-

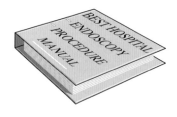

Fig. 1.2 Endoscopy unit practices are collected in a procedure manual.

porting methods—handwritten notes, preprinted forms, free dictation and computer databases.

Eventually all of this documentation (nursing, administrative and endoscopic) will be incorporated in a comprehensive electronic management system. Such a system will substantially reduce the paperwork burden, and increase both efficiency and quality.

EDUCATIONAL RESOURCES

Endoscopy units should offer educational resources for all of its users, including patients, staff and doctors. Clinical staff need a selection of relevant books, atlases, key reprints and journals, and publications of professional societies. Increasingly, many of these materials are available on-line, so that easy internet access should be available. Many organizations produce useful educational videotapes and CD-ROMs and DVDs are increasingly available. In the future some of these tools will be linked directly with endoscopy reporting systems.

Computer simulators are becoming valuable training (and credentialing) tools. Teaching units will need to embrace that technology also.

Patients are also increasingly interested and well served with educational materials. Details are given in Chapter 8.

FURTHER READING

AGA Standards for Office-Based Gastrointestinal Endoscopy Services. *Gastroenterology* 2001; 121: 440–43.

American Society for Gastrointestinal Endoscopy. Establishment of gastrointestinal areas. *Gastrointest Endosc* 1999; 50: 910–12.

Blades EW, Chak A, eds. *Upper Gastrointestinal Endoscopy. Gastrointestinal Endoscopy Clinics of North America*, Vol. 4 (3) (series ed. Sivak MV). Philadelphia: WB Saunders, 1994.

DiMagno EP. Setting up an endoscopy unit. In: Axon, A, ed. *Infection in Endoscopy. Gastrointestinal Endoscopy Clinics of North America*, Vol. 3 (3) (series ed. Sivak MV). Philadelphia: WB Saunders, 1993: 507–71.

Foote MA. *The role of the gastrointestinal assistant.* In: *Gastrointestinal Endoscopy Clinics of North America* (series ed. Sivak MV). Philadelphia: WB Saunders 1994: 523–39.

Quine, MA, Bell, GD, McCloy, RF, Charlton, JE, Devlin, HB, Hopkins, A. Prospective audit of upper gastrointestinal endoscopy in two regions of England; safety and staffing, and sedation methods. *Gut* 1995; 462–7.

Shephard M, Mason J, eds. *Practical Endoscopy.* Chapman & Hall 1997.

2

Equipment

A BRIEF HISTORY

Some older gastroenterologists can remember when endoscopy consisted of rigid metal sigmoidoscopes and esophagoscopes (wielded by thoracic surgeons), and so-called 'semiflexible' gastroscopes. These were metal tubes with a somewhat flexible tip, providing limited views (and no tissue sampling), at considerable discomfort. They were used by only a few enthusiasts in the 1930s through the 1960s. Better gastric visualization was achieved with intragastric cameras, devised by the Japanese because of their focus on gastric cancer. The (British) description of image transmission around bends using fiber-optic bundles led quickly to the development of truly flexible gastroscopes in the USA and then Japan. These entered clinical practice in the mid-1960s. Their popularity was further stimulated by improved visualization, increased tip control, and by the development of a biopsy capability. The latter went some way to providing scientific legitimacy to a technique that was initially shunned by the academic world. Instruments were developed specifically for total upper endoscopy ('pan-endoscopy'), for colonoscopy, and then for duodenoscopy and enteroscopy. More details about the early days of colonoscopy are given in Chapter 6.

Subsequent refinement and the proliferation of therapeutic applications moved endoscopy into the mainstream of gastroenterology, and fueled its enormous expansion worldwide. It is ironic that many academic units in the USA, which initially derided endoscopy, are now largely supported by its financial fruits.

Another important technical breakthrough occurred in the 1980s, with the introduction of video-chip technology. Videoscopes allow the digital image to be displayed conveniently for the endoscopist (no longer poring over the eyepiece), and for the staff and trainees. Also, the image can be stored, processed, analyzed and transmitted anywhere.

Other revolutions are in process now. The transmitting wholly swallowed endoscopy capsule has arrived, and endoscopists are further encroaching on traditional surgical territory with the development of sewing devices. The marriage between endoscopy and computing will produce many more magical new tools. Computer simulation will dramatically change teaching and credentialing.

ENDOSCOPES

Although endoscopes now come in numerous varieties, sizes and applications, they have many common features. They have a control head with valves (buttons) for air insufflation and suction, a flexible shaft carrying the light guide and one or more service channels, and a maneuverable bending section at the tip. An umbilical 'connecting tube' joins the endoscope with the light source and processor, and supplies air and suction (Fig. 2.1). The image is transmitted via a fiber-optic bundle, or electronically from a charge-coupled device (CCD) chip.

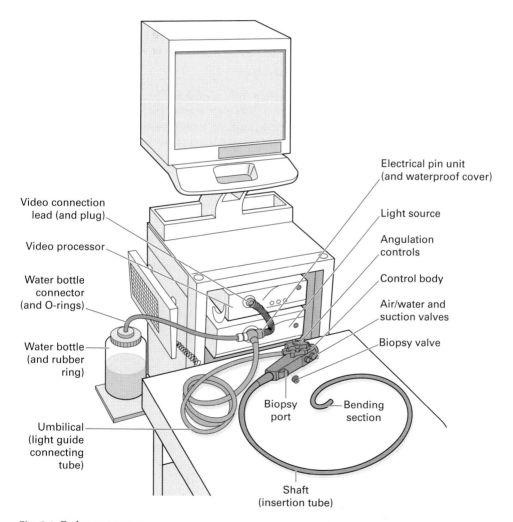

Fig. 2.1 Endoscope system.

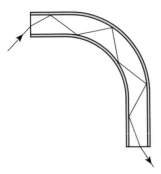

Fig. 2.2 Total internal reflection of light down a glass fiber.

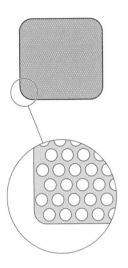

Fig. 2.3 Fiber bundle showing the 'packing fraction' or dead space between fibers.

Fiberscopes

Fiberscopes use optical viewing bundles that contain thousands of fine glass fibers. Light impacting the face of each fiber is transmitted by repeated internal reflections (Fig. 2.2). Faithful transmission of an image depends upon the spatial orientation of the individual fibers being the same at both ends of the bundle (a 'coherent' bundle). Each individual glass fiber is coated with glass of a lower optical density to prevent leakage of light from within the fiber, since the coating does not transmit light. This coating (Fig. 2.2) and the space between the fibers causes a dark 'packing fraction', which is responsible for the fine mesh frequently apparent in the fiber-optic image (Fig. 2.3). For this reason, the image quality of a fiber-optic bundle, though excellent, can never equal that of a rigid lens system.

Video-endoscopes

These are mechanically similar to fiberscopes, but the image is captured with a CCD chip, transmitted electronically, and displayed on a video monitor. Viewing through a monitor has several advantages. The endoscopist does not have to keep his neck bent down to the eyepiece (which can result in 'endoscopist's neck'), and peripheral vision is maintained to appreciate other activities in the room. Other people in the room (including the patient) can watch the video display, and the assistants are more involved in the procedure. Keeping the endoscopist's face away from the biopsy/suction port also reduces the risk of splash contamination.

Individual photo cells (pixels) in the CCD chips can respond only to degrees of light and dark. Color appreciation is arranged by two methods. So-called 'color CCDs' have their pixels arranged under a series of color filter stripes (Fig. 2.4). By contrast,

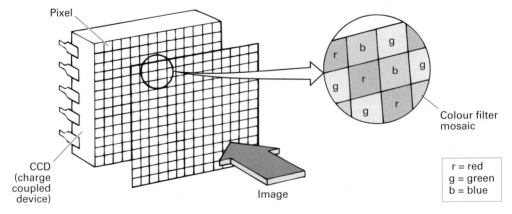

Fig. 2.4 Static red, green and blue filters in the 'color' chip.

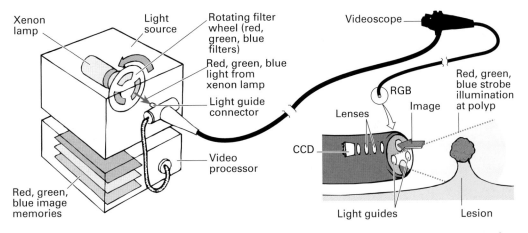

Fig. 2.5 Sequential color illumination.

'black and white CCDs' (or, more correctly, sequential system CCDs) use a rotating color filter wheel to illuminate all of the pixels with primary color strobe-effect lighting (Fig. 2.5). This type of chip can be made smaller, or can give higher resolution, but the system is more expensive because of the additional mechanics and image-processing technology.

Illumination is provided from an external high-intensity source through one or more light-carrying fiber bundles.

Tip control

The distal bending section (10 cm or so) tip of the endoscope is fully deflectable, usually in both planes, up to 180°. Control depends upon pull wires attached at the tip just beneath its outer protective sheath, and passing back through the length of the instrument shaft to the two angulation control wheels (for up/down and right/left movement) on the control head (Fig. 2.6). The wheels incorporate a friction breaking system, so that the tip can be fixed temporarily in any desired position. The instrument shaft is torque stable, so that rotating movements applied to the head are transmitted to the tip—when the shaft is relatively straight. Mechanical angulation controls may soon be replaced by electronic devices.

Instrument channels and valves

The internal anatomy of endoscopes is complex (Fig. 2.7). The shaft incorporates an 'instrumentation' channel extending from the entry 'biopsy port' to the tip of the instrument. Channel sizes vary from about 1 to 5 mm (but usually about 3 mm) depending upon the purpose for which the endoscope was designed (from neonatal examinations to major therapeutic procedures). In

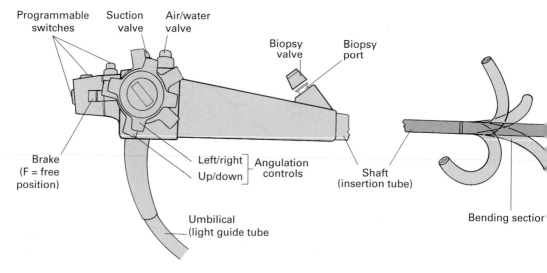

Fig. 2.6 Basic design—control head and bending section.

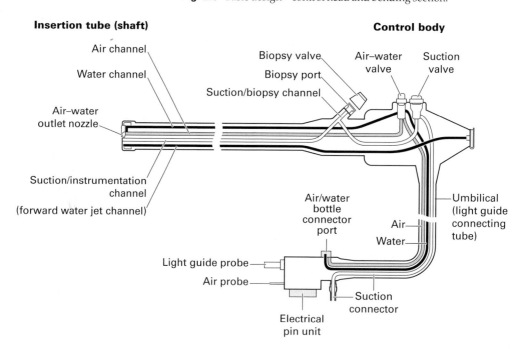

Fig. 2.7 The internal anatomy of a typical endoscope.

some instruments, especially those with lateral-viewing optics, the tip of the channel incorporates a deflectable elevator or bridge (Fig. 2.8), which permits directional control of forceps and other accessories independent of the instrument tip; this elevator is controlled by a further thumb lever. The operating channel is used also for aspirating secretions; an external suction pump is connected to the 'umbilical' of the instrument near to the light source, and suction is diverted into the instrument channel by pressing the suction valve. Another small channel allows passage of air to distend the organ being examined; the air is supplied from a pump in the light source and is controlled by another valve. The air system also pressurizes the water bottle, so that a jet of water can be squirted across the distal lens to clean it.

Different instruments

The endoscopy unit must have a selection of endoscopes for specific applications. They may differ in length, size, stiffness, channel size and number, sophistication and distal lens orientation. Most endoscopies are performed with instruments providing *direct forward vision*, via a wide-angle lens (up to 130°) (Fig. 2.9). However, there are circumstances in which it is preferable to view *laterally*—particularly for ERCP (Fig. 2.8). Oblique and even movable-lens instruments have been developed, but are no longer popular.

The overall diameter of an endoscope is a compromise between engineering ideals and patient tolerance. The shaft must contain and protect many bundles, wires and tubes, all of which are stronger and more efficient when larger (Fig. 2.7). A colonoscope can reasonably approach 15 mm in diameter, but this size is acceptable in the upper gut only for specialized therapeutic instruments.

Routine upper endoscopy is mostly performed with instruments of 8–11 mm diameter. Smaller endoscopes are available; they are better tolerated by all patients and have specific application in children. Some can be passed through the nose rather than the mouth. However, smaller instruments inevitably involve some compromise in durability, image quality, maneuverability, biopsy size, and therapeutic potential.

Several companies now produce a full range of endoscopes at comparable prices. However, light sources and processors produced by different companies are not interchangeable, so that most endoscopy units concentrate for convenience on equipment from a single manufacturer. Endoscopes are delicate, and some breakages are inevitable. Careful maintenance and close communication, repair and back-up arrangements with an efficient company are necessary to maintain an endoscopy service. The quality of the support is often a crucial factor affecting the choice of manufacturer.

ENDOSCOPIC ACCESSORIES

Many devices can be passed through the endoscope channel for diagnostic and therapeutic purposes.

Biopsy forceps consist of a pair of sharpened cups (Fig. 2.10), a spiral metal cable, a pull wire, and a control handle (Fig. 2.11).

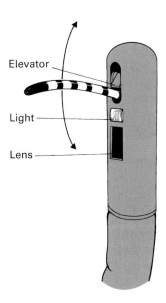

Fig. 2.8 A side-viewer with a deflectable elevator.

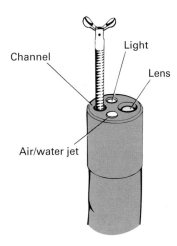

Fig. 2.9 The tip of a forward-viewing endoscope.

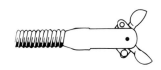

Fig. 2.10 Biopsy cups open.

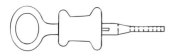

Fig. 2.11 Control handle for forceps.

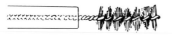

Fig. 2.12 Cytology brush with outer sleeve.

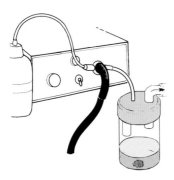

Fig. 2.13 A suction trap to collect fluid specimens.

Their maximum diameter is limited by the size of the operating channel, and the length of the cups by the radius of curvature through which they must pass in the instrument tip. When taking biopsy specimens from a lesion that can only be approached tangentially (e.g. the wall of the esophagus), forceps with a central spike may be helpful; however, these do present a significant puncture hazard for staff.

Cytology brushes have a covering plastic sleeve to protect the specimen during withdrawal (Fig. 2.12).

Needle aspiration devices are also sometimes used for tissue sampling. Similar needles are used for injecting.

Fluid-flushing devices—to provide optical views of lesions, it is sometimes necessary to flush fluids through the operating channel. This can be done with a large syringe or a pulsatile electric pump, with a suitable nozzle inserted into the biopsy port. Some therapeutic instruments have an in-built forward-facing flushing channel at the tip. For more precise aiming, a washing catheter can be passed down the channel to clean specific areas of interest, or to highlight mucosal detail by 'dye spraying' (using a nozzle-tipped catheter).

ANCILLARY EQUIPMENT

Suction traps (fitted temporarily into the suction line) can be used to take samples of intestinal secretions and bile for microbiology, chemistry, and cytology (Fig. 2.13, see also Fig. 7.27).

Biteguards are used to protect the patient's teeth, and also the endoscope from the occasional bite. Some have straps to keep them in place, and oxygen ports.

Overtubes are flexible plastic sleeves that cover the endoscope shaft, and act as a conduit for repeated intubations, or to facilitate therapeutic procedures such as foreign body extraction and hemostasis (Fig. 2.14).

Stretchers/trolleys. Endoscopy is normally performed on a standard transportation stretcher. This should have rails, and preferably allow height adjustment. The ability to tilt the stretcher head down may be helpful in emergencies.

Image documentation. Fiberscopes use specially adapted print cameras. Videoscopes capture images digitally, which can then be enhanced, stored, transmitted and printed. Video sequences can be recorded on tape or digitally.

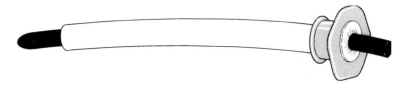

Fig. 2.14 An overtube with biteguard over a rubber lavage tube.

ENERGY SOURCES

Electrosurgical units

Any electrosurgical unit can, if necessary, be used for endoscopic therapy but purpose-built isolated-circuit and 'intelligent' units have major advantages in safety and ease of use. The best electrosurgical units have test circuitry and an automatic warning system or cut-out in case a connection is faulty or the patient plate is not in contact. Electrosurgical units have separate 'cut' and 'coagulate' circuits, which can often be blended to choice. For flexible endoscopy, low-power settings are used (typically 15–50 W). However, in the most advanced units an 'auto-cut' option may be available, which uses an apparently higher power setting but gives good control of tissue heating and cutting, because the system automatically adjusts power output according to initial tissue resistance and increasing resistance during coagulation and desiccation.

In electrosurgery, the type of current is generally less important than the amount of power produced, and other physical factors such as electrode pressure or snare-wire thickness and squeeze are more critical. High settings (high power) of coagulating current provide satisfactory cutting characteristics, whereas units with output not rated directly in watts can be assumed to have 'cut' power output much greater than that of 'coag' at the same setting. The difference in current type used is therefore often illusory. If in doubt, pure coagulating current alone is considered by most expert endoscopists to be safer and more predictable, giving 'slow cook' effect and maximum hemostasis.

Lasers and plasma coagulation

Lasers (particularly the neodymium-YAG and argon lasers) were introduced into endoscopy for treatment of bleeding ulcers, and for tumor ablation, because it seemed desirable to use a 'no touch' technique. However, it has become clear that the same effects can be achieved with much less expensive devices, and that pressure (coaptation) may actually be helpful (for hemostasis).

Argon plasma coagulation (APC) is safer, easier to use and as effective as lasers for most endoscopic purposes. APC electrocoagulates, without tissue contact, by using the electrical conductivity of argon gas—a similar phenomenon to that seen in neon lights. The argon, passed down an electrode catheter (Fig. 2.15a) and energized with an intelligent-circuitry electrosurgical unit and patient plate, ionizes to produce a local plasma arc—like a miniature lightning strike (Fig. 2.15b). The heating effect is inherently superficial (2–3 mm at most, unless current is applied in the same place for many seconds), because tissue coagulation increases resistance and causes the plasma arc to jump elsewhere.

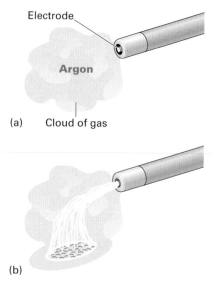

Fig. 2.15 Argon plasma coagulation (APC).

However, APC action alone may be too superficial to debulk a larger lesion, requiring preliminary piecemeal snare-loop removal, with APC to electrocoagulate the base.

Diode and tuned dye lasers are therefore now used only in a few specialist units, largely related to oncology, and have little relevance to ordinary practice.

EQUIPMENT MAINTENANCE

Endoscopes are expensive and complex tools. They should be stored safely, hanging vertically in cupboards through which air can circulate. Care must be taken when carrying instruments, since the optics are easily damaged if left to dangle or knocked against a hard surface. The head, tip and umbilical cord should all be held (Fig. 2.16).

The life of an endoscope is largely determined by the quality of maintenance. Complex accessories (e.g. electrosurgical equipment) must be checked and kept in safe condition. Close collaboration with hospital bioengineering departments and servicing engineers is essential, but most of the work is done by the unit staff. Repairs and maintenance must be properly documented.

Channel blockage

Blockage of the air/water (or suction) channel is one of the most common endoscope problems. Special 'channel flushing devices' are available, allowing separate syringe flushing of the air and water channels; they should be used routinely. When blockage

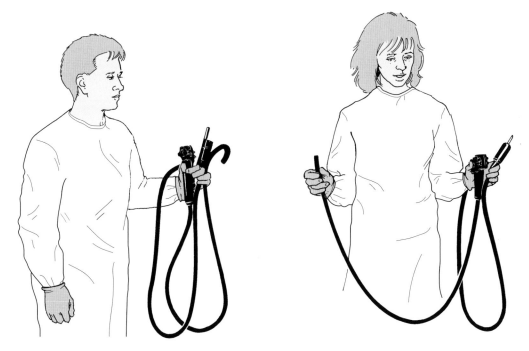

Fig. 2.16 Carry endoscopes carefully to avoid knocks to the optics in the control head and tip.

occurs, the various systems and connections (instrument umbilical, water bottle cap or tube, etc.) must be checked, including the tightness and the presence of rubber O-rings where relevant. It is usually possible to clear the different channels by using the manufacturer's flushing device or a syringe with a suitable soft plastic introducer or micropipette tip. Water can be injected down any channel and, because water is not compressed, more force can be applied than with air. Remember that a small syringe (1–5 mL) generates more pressure than a large one, whereas a large one (50 mL) generates more suction. The air or suction connections at the umbilical, or the water tube within the water bottle can be syringed until water emerges from the instrument tip. Care should be taken to cover or depress the relevant control valves while syringing. Another method for unclogging the suction channel is to remove the valve, and apply suction directly at the port.

INFECTION CONTROL

There is a risk of transmitting infection in the endoscopy unit, from patient to patient, patient to staff, and even from staff to patient. Universal precautions should always be adopted. This means assuming that all patients are somehow infectious, even if there is no objective evidence. Infection control experts and

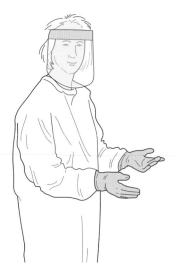

Fig. 2.17 Gowns, gloves and eye protection should be worn.

equipment manufacturers should be welcomed as partners in minimizing infection risk; they should be invited to participate in developing unit policies, and in monitoring their effectiveness, through formal quality control processes. Infection control policies should be written down and understood by all staff.

Staff protection

Staff should be immunized against hepatitis; tuberculosis checks are mandatory in some units. Splashing with body fluids is a risk for staff in contact with patients and instruments. Gowns, gloves and eye protection should be worn for these activities (Fig. 2.17).

Other measures to reduce the risk of infection include:
• frequent hand-washing;
• rigorous use of paper towels when handling soiled accessories;
• putting soiled items directly into a sink or designated area (not on clean surfaces);
• covering skin breaks with a waterproof dressing;
• appropriate disposal of hazardous waste, needles and syringes;
• general maintenance of good hygienic practice throughout the unit.

CLEANING AND DISINFECTION

There are three levels of disinfection.
1 *Sterilization* is required for *critical re-usable accessories*, which enter body cavities, vasculature or penetrate mucous membranes, e.g. biopsy forceps, sclerotherapy needles and sphincterotomes. 'Single-use' disposable items are pre-sterilized.
2 *High-level disinfection* is required for *semicritical accessories*, which come into contact with mucous membranes, e.g. endoscopes and esophageal dilators.
3 *Low-level disinfection* (essentially 'wipe-down') is adequate for *non-critical accessories*, which come into contact with intact skin, e.g. cameras and endoscopic furniture.

Guidelines for the cleaning and disinfection process vary in different countries. They should be determined in each unit (and documented in the procedure manual) after consulting with infection control consultants, equipment manufacturers, and appropriate national advisory bodies. Endoscopists should be fully aware of their local practice, not least because they may be held legally responsible for any untoward event.

All advisory bodies require high-level disinfection of the endoscopes and other equipment shortly after use.

The process must be repeated before reuse if endoscopes lie idle for more than 24 hours, because they gradually become contaminated.

Formal cleaning and disinfection procedures should take place in a purpose-designed area. There should be clearly defined and separated clean and dirty areas, multiple worktops, double sinks and a separate hand washbasin, endoscopic reprocessors (washing machines) and an ultrasound cleaner. An appropriately placed fume hood is also desirable.

Mechanical cleaning

The first and vitally important task in the disinfection process is to clean the endoscope and all of its channels, to remove all blood, secretions and debris. Disinfectants cannot penetrate organic material.

Initial cleaning must be done immediately after the endoscope is removed from the patient.

• Wipe down with a cloth soaked in enzymatic detergent.
• Suck water and enzymatic detergent through the biopsy channel, alternating with air, until the solution is visibly clean.
• Flush the air/water channel with the manufacturer's flushing device or by depressing the air/water button while occluding the water bottle attachment at the light source and holding the tip of the scope under water. This should be continued until vigorous bubbling is seen.
• Attach the cap designed to protect the electrical connections, and transfer the scope (in protective packaging to avoid contamination) to the designated cleaning area.
• Test the scope for leaks, particularly in the bending section, by pressurizing it with the leak-testing device.
• Remove all valves and biopsy caps.
• Totally immerse the instrument in warm water and neutral detergent. Wash the outside of the instrument thoroughly with a soft cloth.
• Brush the distal end with a soft toothbrush, paying particular attention to the air/water outlet jet and any bridge/elevator.
• Clean the biopsy channel opening and suction port using the cleaning brush provided. Pass a clean brush suitable for the instrument and channel size through the suction channel until it emerges clean (at least three times), cleaning the brush itself each time before reinsertion. Remove the suction button, and pass the cleaning brush through the suction channel opening and down the shaft until it emerges from the distal end, at least three times. Pass the cleaning brush from the suction channel opening in the other direction, through the umbilical, until it emerges from the suction connector at least three times. Repeat the process for all the channels.
• Place the endoscope into a reprocessor to complete cleaning and disinfection (or continue manually).

• Clean all instrument accessories equally scrupulously, including the air/water and suction valves, water bottles and the cleaning brushes.

Disinfection

After thorough cleaning:
• attach the manufacturer's cleaning adapter to the suction, biopsy and air/water channels;
• flush each channel with detergent fluid ensuring that it emerges from the distal end of each channel;
• confirm that all air is expelled from the channels. Soak the instrument in the chosen disinfectant for the recommended contact time.

Disinfectants

Glutaraldehyde is the most popular agent. It can destroy viruses and bacteria within 4 min, is non-corrosive (for the endoscopes), and has a low surface tension, which aids penetration. Most advisory authorities recommend a 20-minute soak time in glutaraldehyde for standard situations, assuming adequate precleaning. More prolonged soaking may be required in cases of known or suspected mycobacterial disease. The instrument accessories (valves, water bottles, etc.) are also soaked.

Glutaraldehyde does carry the risk of sensitization, and can cause severe dermatitis, sinusitis or asthma among exposed staff. The risk increases with increasing levels and duration of exposure. Heavy domestic-grade rubber gloves should be worn when using glutaraldehyde since normal thin medical glove material is permeable to it, and goggles and/or a face mask can protect against splashes. Closed system reprocessors and fume hoods/extraction fans are important. Reprocessors should be self-disinfecting. The concentration of disinfectant should be monitored.

Alcohol, peracetic acid, chlorine dioxide, Sterox and other agents have also been used for endoscope disinfection.

A *sterile water supply* (special filters may be needed) helps to reduce the risk of nosocomial infections, such as *Pseudomonas*.

Rinsing, drying and storing

Following disinfection, reprocessors rinse the instruments internally and externally to remove all traces of disinfectant, using the all-channel irrigator. The air, water and suction channels are perfused with 70% alcohol and dried with forced air before storage. This must be done manually if reprocessors are not used. Bacteria multiply in a moist environment, and the importance of drying instruments after disinfection cannot be overemphasized. Instruments should be hung vertically in a well-ventilated cupboard.

Accessory devices

Diagnostic and therapeutic devices (such as biopsy forceps) are critical accessories, and must be sterile. Many are now disposable. Reusable accessories are autoclaved or gas sterilized.

Quality control

Records should be kept of the disinfection process for every endoscope, including who cleaned it, when, and how. Routine bacteriological surveillance of automatic disinfectors and endoscopes is recommended. This allows early detection of serious contaminating organisms such as *Pseudomonas* and atypical mycobacteria. Routine surveillance also allows the early detection of otherwise unrecognizable internal channel damage, reprocessing protocol errors, as well as any water and environmental contamination problems. Surveillance of duodenoscopes is particularly recommended because of the greater potential clinical impact of serious infections at ERCP.

The spectre of prion-related disease may be raised in patients with degenerative neurological symptoms. Since prion proteins are not inactivated by heat or current disinfection regimes, disposable accessories should be used with a back-up endoscope reserved for such suspect patients. Lymphoid tissue is a particular risk, so many units now advise against routine ileal biopsies, particularly of Peyer's patches, for fear of potential prion contamination of the instrument channels.

Remember, although most of the cleaning, disinfection and maintenance activities are normally and appropriately delegated to the staff, it is the endoscopist who is responsible for ensuring that his equipment is safe to use. Endoscopists should know how to complete the process themselves, especially in some emergency situations where the usual endoscopy nurses unfortunately may not be available.

FURTHER READING

Alvarado CJ, Mark R. APIC guidelines for infection prevention and control in flexible endoscopy. *Am J Infect Control* 2000; 28: 138–55.

American Society for Gastrointestinal Endoscopy. *Monitoring Equipment for Endoscopy.* ASGE Technology Assessment Status Evaluation. Manchester: American Society for Gastrointestinal Endoscopy, 1994.

American Society for Gastrointestinal Endoscopy. Infection control during gastrointestinal endoscopy: guidelines for clinical application. *Gastrointest Endosc* 1999; 49: 836–41.

Axon ATR, ed. *Infection in Endoscopy. Gastrointestinal Endoscopy Clinics of North America*, Vol. 3(3) (series ed. Sivak MV). Philadelphia: WB Saunders, 1993.

British Endoscopy Committee Working Party. Cleaning and disinfection of equipment for gastrointestinal endoscopy: report of a working party of the British Society of Gastroenterology Endoscopy Committee. *Gut* 1998; 42: 585–93.

Carr-Locke DL, Conn MI, Faigel DO *et al*. Technology status evaluation: personal protective equipment. *Gastrointest Endosc* 1999; 49: 854–7.

Cowen A. Infection and endoscopy: patient to patient transmission. In: Axon, ATR, ed. *Infection in Endoscopy. Gastrointestinal Endoscopy Clinics of North America*, Vol. 3(3) (series ed. Sivak MV). Philadelphia: WB Saunders, 1993: 483–96.

DiMarino AJ Jr, Leung J, Ravich W *et al*. Reprocessing of flexible gastrointestinal endoscopes. *Gastrointest Endosc* 1996; 43: 540–6.

DiMarino J, Erage T, Leung J. Reprocessing of flexible gastrointestinal endoscopes. *Gastrointest Endosc* 1996; 43: 540–6.

Gruber M, Seebald C, Byrd R, Tomasulo V, Mahl T. Electrocautery and patients with implanted cardiac devices. *Gastroenterol Nurs* 1995; 38: 49–53.

Kimmey MB, Al-Kawas FH, Burnett DA. Electrocautery use in patients with implanted cardiac devices. *Gastrointest Endosc* 1994; 40 (6): 794–5.

Kimmey MB, Al-Kawas FH, Gannan RM *et al*. Technology Status Evaluation: disposable endoscopic accessories. *Gastrointest Endosc* 1995; 42: 618–19 (and 1993; 39: 878–80).

Kimmey MB, Burnett DA, Carr-Locke DL *et al*. Transmission of infection by gastrointestinal endoscopy. *Gastrointest Endosc* 1993; 39: 885–8.

Nelson DB, Bosco JJ, Curtis WD. Automatic endoscopic reprocessors. *Gastrointest Endosc* 1999; 50: 925–7.

Nelson DB. Transmission of infection during gastrointestinal endoscopy. *Clin Update Am Soc for Gastrointestinal Endoscopy* 2002; 9 (3): 1–3.

Nelson DB, Bosco JJ, Curtis WD *et al*. ASGE Technology Status Evaluation Report: automatic endoscope reprocessors. *Gastrointest Endosc* 1990; 50: 925–7.

O'Connor HJ. Risk of sepsis in endoscopic procedures. In: Axon, ATR, ed. *Infection in Endoscopy. Gastrointestinal Endoscopy Clinics of North America*, Vol. 3(3) (series ed. Sivak MV). Philadelphia: WB Saunders, 1993; 459–68.

Rutala WA. APIC guidelines for selection and use of disinfectants. *Am J Infect Control* 1990; 18: 99.

Rutala WA, Weber DJ. Creutzfeldt–Jakob disease. Recommendations for disinfection and sterilization. *Clin Infect Dis* 2001; 32: 1348–56.

World Health Organization. *WHO Infection Control Guidelines for Transmissible Spongiform Encephalopathies*. WHO/CDS/CSR/APH/2000.3. Geneva: WHO, 1999.

Zeroske J. Practical disinfection technique. In: Axon, ATR, ed. *Infection in Endoscopy. Gastrointestinal Endoscopy Clinics of North America*, Vol. 3(3) (series ed. Sivak MV). Philadelphia: WB Saunders, 1993.

Patient Care

Skilled endoscopists can now reach every part of the digestive tract, and its appendages such as the biliary tree and pancreas. It is possible to take specimens from all of these areas, and to treat many of their afflictions. Many patients have benefited greatly from endoscopy. Unfortunately, in some cases it may be unhelpful, and can even result in severe complications. There are also some hazards for the staff. The goal must be to maximize the benefits and minimize the risks. We need to be experts, working for good indications on patients who are fully prepared and protected, with skilled assistants, and using optimum equipment. The basic principles are similar for all areas of gastrointestinal (GI) endoscopy, recognizing that there are specific circumstances where the risks are greater, including therapeutic and emergency procedures.

Endoscopy is normally part of a comprehensive evaluation by a gastroenterologist or other digestive specialist. It is mostly used electively in the practice environment, or hospital outpatient clinic, but sometimes may be needed in any part of a healthcare facility (e.g. Emergency Room, Intensive Care Unit, Operating Room). Sometimes, endoscopists offer an 'open access' service, where the initial clinical assessment and continuing care are performed by another physician.

In all of these situations it is the responsibility of endoscopists to ensure that the potential benefits exceed the potential risks, and personally to perform the necessary evaluations to make appropriate recommendations for their patients.

The following sections refer primarily to upper endoscopy. Issues specific to colonoscopy are covered in Chapters 6 and 7.

INDICATIONS FOR UPPER ENDOSCOPY

Upper endoscopy is now the primary tool for evaluating the esophagus, stomach and duodenum. It may be used for many reasons.

Broadly speaking, the goal may be:
1 To make a diagnosis in the presence of suggestive symptoms (e.g. dyspepsia, heartburn, dysphagia, anorexia, weight loss, hematemesis, anemia).
2 To clarify the status of a known disease (e.g. varices, Barrett's esophagus).
3 To take target specimens (e.g. duodenal biopsy for malabsorption).

4 To screen for malignancy and premalignancy in patients judged to be at increased risk of neoplasia (e.g. familial adenomatous polyposis).
5 To perform therapy (e.g. hemostasis, dilatation, polypectomy, foreign body removal, tube placement, gastrostomy).

Several indications may be combined, for example 1 and 5 (in acute bleeding), or 2 and 5 (e.g. retreatment of known varices).

PATIENT PREPARATION

Patients must be carefully prepared for their procedures, both mentally and physically, to ensure safety, comfort and success.

Mental preparation

Mental preparation includes explanation of the endoscopy process, i.e. the practical issues of what exactly will happen, with reassurance about common concerns.

Informed consent is a medico-legal requirement in most institutions. It describes the essential process of communication, education and understanding—not just a paper form to be signed. Patients are entitled to be fully informed of the reasons why a procedure is recommended, its expected benefits, the potential risks, its limitations and the alternatives. Printed brochures can facilitate this education process (Fig. 3.1), and should be given (or sent) to patients well in advance of the procedures, so that they can be studied carefully and digested. Suitable brochures are available from national organizations, and on web sites from expert centers (e.g. www.ddc.musc.edu). They can be adapted or developed for local conditions. Some centers use videotapes and web-based instructional materials. Patients must be given the opportunity to ask questions of the endoscopist before being invited to confirm their understanding and agreement to the procedure by signing the consent form.

Physical preparation

Physical preparation includes taking nothing by mouth for about six hours (usually overnight), changing into a loose-fitting gown, and undergoing a series of medical checks and actions to optimize the safety of the intervention. This involves a general medical review, including vital signs and cardiopulmonary status, and attention to many details concerning risks and risk reduction. Intravenous access should be established, preferably in the right arm or hand. Spectacles and dentures are removed, and stored safely.

Preparation specific for colonoscopy is covered in Chapter 6.

Upper Endoscopy

Upper endoscopy is a test that lets your doctor see the lining of your upper digestive system and often make a diagnosis or treat. The upper digestive system includes the food tube (esophagus), stomach and the first part of the small intestine (duodenum).

Upper endoscopy is the best way to find swelling (inflammation), ulcers or tumors of the upper digestive system.

Upper endoscopy can be used to treat some conditions present in the upper digestive system. Growths (polyps) and swallowed objects can be removed. Narrow areas can be stretched. Bleeding can be treated.

What is an Endoscope?

An endoscope is a long, narrow, flexible tube containing a tiny light and camera at one end.
This camera carries pictures of your upper digestive tract to a television screen. The doctor and nurse can see your esophagus, stomach, and small intestine better on this monitor. The pictures can also be recorded and printed.

How Do I Prepare?

Do not eat or drink for 6 hours before your test. Your stomach must be empty.

Tell your doctor if you...
• have any allergies, heart or lung problems.
• are or think you may be pregnant.
• have had endoscopy in the past and if you had problems with the medicines used.
• take antibiotics before having dental work.

If you take medicine to thin your blood, (i.e. heparin or coumadin) or aspirin compounds tell your doctor. In general, you must stop taking these pills for several days, but in some cases you may continue to take them.

If you are a diabetic, please ask your doctor if you should take your insulin and/or pills before your test.

You may take blood pressure and heart medicine as usual the morning of your test.

If you take pills in the morning, drink only a small sip of water to help you swallow.

Do not take any antacids.

Bring with you all prescription and over-the-counter medicines you are taking.

Bring with you all medical records and X-ray films that relate to your current problem.

Make sure an adult can take you home. The medicines used during the procedure will not wear off for several hours. You will NOT be able to drive. If you travel by public transportation, such as by bus, van or taxi, you will still need an adult to ride home with you.

If you come alone, (and need medicines for sedation), your test will have to be rescheduled.

Fig. 3.1 Patient education brochure. (*Continued overleaf.*)

What Will Happen During My Upper Endoscopy?

1.　　　When you come for the Upper Endoscopy, the doctor will talk to you about the test and answer any questions you have. You should know why you are having an Upper Endoscopy and understand the treatment options and possible risks.

2.　　　You will put on a hospital gown. You will be asked to remove any eye glasses, contact lenses or dentures. An IV will be started and blood may be drawn for lab studies. You may receive antibiotics through the IV at this time.

3.　　　You will be asked to sign a consent form which gives the doctor your permission to do the test.

4.　　　You will be taken by stretcher to the procedure room. The nurse will help you get into the correct position, usually on your side, and make you comfortable. A medicine will be sprayed onto the back of your throat to make it numb. The medicine may taste unpleasant but it will stop any coughing during the test and the taste will go away quickly. A plastic guard will be placed in your mouth to protect your teeth during the test.

5.　　　A blood pressure cuff will be put on your arm or leg. A small clip will be put on your finger. These will let the nurse check your blood pressure and heart rate frequently during the test.

6.　　　If you require sedation, you will be given medicine through the IV. When you are relaxed and sleepy, the doctor will place a thin, flexible endoscope through the mouth guard and into your mouth. The endoscope has a small video camera on the end that lets the doctor see the inside of your esophagus.

7.　　　The doctor will ask you to swallow. When you swallow, the endoscope will gently move down your esophagus, the same way food goes down when you are eating. You may feel like gagging, but you should not feel any pain. The endoscope will not interfere with your breathing.

8.　　　The doctor will guide the endoscope through your stomach and into your small intestine. This will allow the doctor to see the lining of your upper digestive system and treat any problems that may be found.

9.　　　When the test is done, the doctor will slowly take out the endoscope. Your Upper Endoscopy will last between 5 and 20 minutes.

What Will Happen Afterwards?

1.　　　You will be taken to the recovery area. Your blood pressure and heart rate are watched while you rest.

2.　　　If you have not needed medicines for sedation, you will be able to leave quickly and resume normal activities. After removing your IV, the nurse will give you written instructions to follow when you go home. If you have any questions, please ask. The doctor will talk to you about your test before you leave.

3.　　　If you needed medicines for sedation, your reflexes and judgment will be slow, even if you feel awake. You will NOT be allowed to leave unless an adult takes you home. Do not drive, operate machinery, sign legal documents or make important decisions. Do not drink alcohol or take sleeping or nerve pills.

Fig. 3.1 (*Continued.*)

4.   If treatments were done during your test, you may need to be observed overnight in hospital.

5.   If specimens were taken at your endoscopy, the results will be sent to you and the doctor who is providing your continuing care.

6.   You may feel bloated and pass gas. This is normal and will go away in a few hours. Your throat may be a little sore.

You may resume your regular diet and medications after the procedure.

What are the Risks?

Upper Endoscopy is usually simple, but there are some risks, especially when treatments are done during the test.

A tender lump may form where the IV was placed. You will need to call your doctor if redness, pain or swelling in this hand or arm lasts for more than two days.

The medicines may make you sick. You may have nausea, vomiting, hives, dry mouth, or a reddened face and neck.

Severe problems occur in less than one case in 500. These include chest and heart difficulties, bleeding, or tearing (perforation) of the digestive system. If any of these problems happen, you will have to stay in the hospital. Surgery may be needed.

Your doctor will discuss these risks with you.

Call the Doctor if You....

• have severe pain.
• vomit.
• pass or vomit blood.
• have chills and fever above 101 degrees.

If you have any problems, call your specialist. If it is after regular business hours, page the 'GI Doctor on Call' through the paging operator at ....
This information is provided as an educational service of the ......
The content is limited and is not a substitute for professional medical care.

Fig. 3.1 (*Continued.*)

RISKS AND UNPLANNED EVENTS (COMPLICATIONS)

The vast majority of routine upper endoscopy procedures go according to plan. But, there are exceptions. These may best be generally categorized as 'unplanned events' (or adverse events), since many are relatively trivial (e.g. the need for analgesia reversal during a procedure, or the appearance of tenderness at an infusion site). All deviations from the expected plan of care should be documented, so that quality improvement processes can be applied.

The term 'complication' has unfortunate medico-legal connotations, so its use should be restricted to unplanned events of a certain defined level of severity. Over 10 years ago a group interested in the outcomes of ERCP defined a *complication* as an unplanned event that requires the patient to be admitted to hospital, or to stay longer than expected, or to undergo other interventions. This means that we do not count in complication statistics any deviation that occurs during a procedure that is not obvious to the patient afterwards (e.g. transient bleeding).

Levels of severity

Complications can vary from relatively minor to life-threatening, so it is necessary to have some measure of severity. The same consensus group recommended using the degree of patient 'disturbance' to stratify complications:
- *Mild*—events requiring hospitalization of 1–3 days.
- *Moderate*—hospital stay of 4–9 days.
- *Severe*—stay more than 10 days, or the need for surgery, or intensive care.
- *Fatal*—death attributable to the procedure.

Attribution of delayed events can be contentious. For example, do we count a fatal myocardial infarction if it occurs 3 weeks after endoscopy? Probably not, but what if it occurs only 7 (or 2) days afterwards, especially if the patient had been advised to stop antiplatelet medications?

Timing of events

Unplanned events can occur before the endoscope is introduced (e.g. reaction to antibiotics or other preparation medication), during the procedure (e.g. dysrhythmia, hypoxia), immediately afterwards (e.g. pain due to perforation), or they may be delayed for days or weeks (e.g. delayed bleeding or aspiration pneumonia). Keeping track of events that occur after patients leave the unit is a challenge. Some units have instituted routine follow-up phone calls. As its use spreads, e-mail will have application.

Endoscopy databases should capture all such events, and allow attribution options.

Complication rates

The problems of definition and data collection make it difficult to quote meaningful global statistics about the risks of endoscopy. Large surveys suggest that the chance of suffering a severe complication (such as perforation or cardiopulmonary dysfunction) after routine upper endoscopy is less than one in 500 cases. The risks are higher in the elderly and acutely ill, and during therapeutic and emergency procedures. Inexperience, oversedation and overconfidence are important factors.

Specific events

• *Hypoxia* should be detected early by careful nursing surveillance aided by pulse oximetry. Sometimes it is necessary only to ask the patient to breathe more deeply, and to provide oxygen supplementation. Reversal agents may be necessary.
• *Pulmonary aspiration* is probably commoner than recognized. The risk is greater in patients with retained food residue (e.g. achalasia, pyloric stenosis), and in those with active bleeding.
• *Bleeding* may occur—during and after endoscopy—from existing lesions (e.g. varices), or due to endoscopic manipulation (biopsy, polypectomy) or, occasionally, due to retching from a Mallory–Weiss tear. The risk of bleeding is greater in patients with coagulopathy, and in those taking anticoagulants and (possibly) antiplatelet agents.
• *Perforation* is the most feared complication of upper endoscopy. It is rare, but most commonly occurs in the neck, and is more frequent in elderly patients, perhaps in the presence of a Zenker's diverticulum. The risk is minimized by gentle endoscope insertion under direct vision. Perforation beyond the cricopharyngeus is extremely unusual in patients who are not undergoing therapeutic techniques such as stricture dilatation, polypectomy or mucosal resection. Perforation at colonoscopy is discussed in Chapter 7.
• *Cardiac dysrhythmias* are extremely rare, and require prompt recognition and expert treatment.
• *Intravenous (IV) site problems.* Many patients have discomfort at the site of their intravenous infusion; local thrombosis is not unusual or dangerous, but evidence of spreading inflammation should be treated promptly and seriously.
• *Infection.* Endoscopes (and accessories) are potential vehicles for the transmission of infection from patient to patient (e.g. *Helicobacter pylori*, salmonellas, hepatitis, mycobacteria). This risk should be eliminated by assiduous attention to detail in cleaning and disinfection. Endoscopy can provoke bacteremia, especially

during therapeutic procedures such as dilatation. This may be dangerous in patients who are immunocompromised, and in some with diseased heart valves and prostheses. Endoscopy-induced endocarditis is extremely rare, but antibiotic prophylaxis is advised in certain circumstances (see below).

ASSESSING AND REDUCING RISKS

Endoscopists are obliged to balance the potential risks against the expected benefits before recommending procedures. Knowledge of the risks determines the necessary precautions.

Certain comorbidities and medications clearly increase the risk of endoscopic procedures. A *checklist* should be used to ensure that all of the issues have been addressed. Some of this information must be obtained when the procedure is scheduled, since action is required days ahead of the procedure (e.g. adjusting anticoagulants, stopping aspirin, etc.). Other aspects are dealt with when the patient arrives in the preprocedure area.

• *Cardiac and pulmonary disease.* Patients with recent myocardial infarction, unstable angina or hemodynamic instability are obviously at risk from any intervention. Expert advice should be sought from cardiologists. Endoscopy can be performed in patients with pacemakers and artificial implantable defibrillators—but the latter must be deactivated (with a supplied magnet) if diathermy is performed. Anesthetic supervision is essential if endoscopy is needed in such patients, and in others with respiratory insufficiency.

• *Coagulation disorders.* Patients with a known bleeding diathesis or coagulation disorder should have the situation normalized as far as possible before endoscopy (particularly if biopsy or polypectomy is likely). Anticoagulants can be stopped ahead of time, and (if clinically necessary) replaced by heparin for the period of the procedure, and early recovery. Certain antiplatelet drugs may need to be stopped also. There is little evidence that aspirin and non-steroidal anti-inflammatory drugs (NSAIDs) increase the risk of endoscopic procedures. However, it is common practice to ask about these drugs, and to recommend that they be discontinued for five days before endoscopic procedures.

• *Sedation issues.* Nervous patients and others who have had prior problems with sedation can pose challenges for safe endoscopy. If in doubt, use anesthesia.

• *Endocarditis.* The risk of developing endocarditis after upper endoscopy procedures is extremely small, and there is no evidence that antibiotic prophylaxis is beneficial. However, most experts recommend prophylaxis for patients deemed to be at increased risk for endocarditis (especially those with artificial valves, previous proven endocarditis, recent vascular prostheses and systemic–pulmonary shunts), particularly when they are undergoing procedures known to provoke bacteremia (e.g.

esophageal dilatation). Recommendations are made by national organizations (Table 3.1). The local policy should be documented in the endoscopy unit policy manual.

The ASA score is used in many units to describe broad categories of fitness for procedures and sedation (Table 3.2). Many recommend anesthesia assistance for patients with ASA scores of 3 or greater.

Endoscopies	Patient status	Regime	Alternative in case of allergy
All	Prosthetic valve Prior endocarditis Systemic-pulmonary shunts Vascular graft <1 yr	ampicillin 1 g + gentamicin 1.5 mg/kg IV (max 80 mg) + amoxicillin 500 g po 6 h post	vancomycin 1 g over 1 h + gentamicin 1.5 mg/kg IV (max 80 mg)
All	Immunocompromised (neutrophils <1000, or transplant)	cefotaxime 2 g IV	clindamycin 900 mg IV and aztreonam 1 g IV
Variceal treatment	Cirrhosis with ascites	ofloxacin 200 mg IV over 1 h then 200 mg 12 hourly	—
PEG	All patients	cefazolin 1 g IV	vancomycin 1 g IV over 1 h

Table 3.1 Antibiotic prophylaxis: policy at the Medical University of South Carolina. This is based on guidelines from the American Heart Association and ASGE. Physician discretion is advised for other cardiac lesions (rheumatic valvular heart disease, acquired valvular dysfunction, mitral valve prolapse with insufficiency, hypertrophic cardiomyopathy, congenital malformations) and in patients having sclerotherapy or esophageal dilation. Special circumstances may justify other approaches. The final decision and responsibility rests with the endoscopist in each case.

Classification	Description	Example
Class I	Healthy patient	
Class II	Mild systemic disease—no functional limitations	Controlled hypertension, diabetes
Class III	Severe systemic disease—definite functional limitation	Brittle diabetic, frequent angina, myocardial infarction
Class IV	Severe systemic disease with acute, unstable symptoms	Recent myocardial infarction, congestive heart failure, acute renal failure, uncontrolled active asthma
Class V	Severe systemic disease with imminent risk of death	

Table 3.2 ASA classification—anesthesia risk classes.

MONITORING

Although the endoscopist has overall responsibility, the endoscopy nurse is the practical guardian of the patient's safety and comfort. For simple procedures, the nurse may also be responsible for assisting the endoscopist (e.g. with biopsy sampling). Nursing surveillance should be supplemented with monitoring devices, at least for pulse rate, blood pressure and oxygen saturation. Continuous supplemental oxygen is commonly used in many units. Some argue that this may mask hypoventilation, which is better detected by monitoring of carbon dioxide (capnography). Electrocardiographic monitoring is desirable for any patient with cardiac problems, and for prolonged complex procedures. Emergency drugs and equipment must be available nearby, and the endoscopist should be trained in resuscitation and life support.

Sedation and other medications are given by the endoscopist, or by the nurse under supervision. The nurse should document this process carefully, along with the patient's vital signs, monitoring data, and the patient's response.

Continuous intravenous access must be maintained.

MEDICATIONS AND SEDATION PRACTICE

Sedation practice varies widely throughout the world. In many countries, most routine (diagnostic) upper endoscopy is performed without any sedation, using only pharyngeal anesthesia. Avoiding sedation has obvious advantages in terms of safety and fast recovery (e.g. patients can drive themselves home). However, many Western patients expect and receive some degree of sedation/analgesia. Chapter 7 includes some discussion about sedation in general, and specifically for colonoscopy.

'Conscious sedation' is intended to make unpleasant procedures tolerable for patients, while maintaining their ability to self-ventilate, maintain a clear airway, and to respond to physical stimulation and verbal commands. Endoscopists giving conscious sedation must be fully familiar with the techniques. Many centers mandate specific training, and credentialing, for 'conscious sedation', supervised by anesthesiology. In contrast to conscious sedation, 'deep sedation' is present when the patient cannot be easily aroused, and may be accompanied by partial or complete loss of protective reflexes, including the ability to maintain a patent airway. This level of sedation requires anesthesiologist supervision.

Sedating/analgesic agents	Initial IV dose	Onset	Duration of effect
midazolam	0.5–2 mg	1–5 min	1–2 h
diazepam	1–5 mg	1–5 min	2–6 h
meperidine	25–50 mg	5–10 min	2–4 h
fentanyl	50–100 µg	1 min	20–60 min
diphenhydramine	10–50 mg	1–10 min	2–6 h
droperidol	1–5 mg	5–10 min	2–4 h
Reversal agents			
flumazenil (for benzodiazepines)	0.1–0.2 mg	30–60 s	30–60 min
naloxone (for opioids)	0.2–0.4 mg (IV & IM)	1–2 min	45 min

Table 3.3 Commonly used medication agents. For sedation purposes 25–50% increments of the initial dose can be administered every 5–10 minutes. Dosages should be adjusted according to patient age, body weight, medical history and concomitant drug use.

Sedation/analgesia agents (Table 3.3)

Anxiolytics

Short-acting benzodiazepines are commonly administered by slow intravenous injection/titration. Midazolam (Versed®) is given in an initial dose of 0.5–2.0 mg, with increments of 0.5–1 mg every 5 minutes, to a maximum of about 5 mg. Doses are determined by the patient's age, weight, medical and drug history, and by the response. Diazepam (Valium®, or in emulsion as Diazemuls®) can be used instead.

Narcotics

Narcotic analgesics are often given with benzodiazepines, but the combination increases the risk of respiratory depression. Pethidine (meperidine) is given in an initial dose of 25–50 mg, with increments of 25 mg up to a maximum of 100–150 mg. Fentanyl (Sublimaze®) is a more potent opioid analgesic, with increased risk of respiratory depression. It is useful in patients intolerant to meperidine.

Droperidol (in increments of 0.5 mg up to about 5 mg) may be a useful adjunct in patients who are difficult to sedate, particularly those with agitation, or a history of heavy alcohol or drug misuse. Hypotension can occur. Recently, reports of some cardiac dysrhythmias have led to a recommendation not to use droperidol when the QT interval is prolonged.

Antagonists

Meperidine® can be reversed by naloxone, given both intramuscularly (IM) and intravenously (IV). Benzodiazepines are reversed by flumazenil, given by slow IV injection. Both antagonists have shorter half-lives than the drugs they antagonize.

Anesthesia

Although the vast majority of standard upper endoscopy procedures can be performed with endoscopist-directed sedation (or with no sedation), there are circumstances where the presence of an anesthesiologist is helpful, and some in which full anesthesia is required. Examples include young children, heavy drinkers, patients who are difficult to sedate, and patients with high-risk cardiopulmonary status. Propofol (Diprivan®) is a useful short-acting anesthesia agent that seems ideal for endoscopy procedures. In most centers and countries this can be given only by anesthesiologists.

Numerous other sedation/anesthesia practices have also been tested and used, for example patient-controlled nitrous oxide, and acupuncture.

Other medications

Pharyngeal anesthesia (given by spray) is used in many units. Avoid asking the patient to say 'ah', since this exposes the larynx also to anesthesia, and may suppress the cough reflex. Some avoid local anesthesia when using sedation, believing that it may increase the risk of aspiration.

Excessive intestinal contraction can be suppressed with intravenous injections of *glucagon* (increments of 0.25 mg up to 2 mg), or *hyoscine butylbromide* (Buscopan®) 20–40 mg, in countries where it is available.

Silicone-containing emulsions can be given to suppress foaming in the stomach—either swallowed before the procedure, or injected down the endoscope channel.

RECOVERY AND DISCHARGE

After the endoscope is removed, the assisting nurse checks on the status of the patient, and then transfers care to the recovery area staff. Monitoring is continued until the patient is fully awake, usually 20–30 minutes after standard sedation. A longer period of observation is necessary after general anesthesia.

A drink is appreciated after the sedation and any pharyngeal anesthesia has worn off. When established discharge criteria are met, the patient dresses and is taken to an interview area to discuss the findings and further care. Endoscopy is not complete until the patient has been counseled about the findings, their implications, and resulting plans. If sedation has been given, it is essential that this process takes place in the presence of an accompanying person, because of the potential for significant delayed amnesia.

Discharge instructions should be given in writing, including details of:

- Resumption of diet and activities.
- Medications to be restarted, stopped and commenced.
- Further appointments.
- How biopsy results will be communicated.
- Symptoms to report (and who to contact):
  - severe pain;
  - distension;
  - fever;
  - vomiting or passing blood.

Some units also print out and provide patient education materials relevant to the specific endoscopic findings. This service will become automatic with fully integrated electronic endoscopy reporting and management systems.

RISK MANAGEMENT

Careful attention to all of these details will help to ensure that most procedures will go smoothly, but unplanned events do occur even in the best of hands and environments.

Endoscopists and the staff naturally feel badly when things 'go wrong', especially when they are severe or life-threatening. It is very important to prepare for and manage these situations appropriately. Firstly, the well-informed patient (and relatives) has been told and should know that bad things can happen. This is an integral and important part of the communication and consent process. So, it is appropriate and correct to address complications in that spirit.

For example: 'It looks like we have a perforation here. We discussed that as a remote possibility beforehand, and I'm sorry that it has occurred. This is what I think we should do'.

Your distress is understandable and worthy, and you need to be sympathetic, but it is important also to be professional and matter of fact. Excessive apologies may give the impression that some avoidable mishap has occurred. Never, never attempt to cover up the facts. Document what has happened and communicate widely—with the patient, interested relatives, referring doctors, supervisors, and your risk management office.

Act quickly. Delay in managing complications is foolish and can be dangerous both medically and legally. Get appropriate radiographs and lab studies, expert advice, and a surgical opinion (from a surgeon who understands the issues) for anything that might remotely require surgical intervention. Sometimes it may be wise to offer transfer of the patient to a colleague or to a larger center, but, if this happens, try to keep in touch, and to show continuing interest and concern. Patients (and relatives) who feel abandoned are often litigious.

The American Society for Gastrointestinal Endoscopy (ASGE) has excellent publications on these issues (http://www.asge.org).

FURTHER READING

American Society for Gastrointestinal Endoscopy. *Monitoring Equipment for Endoscopy*. ASGE Technology Assessment Status Evaluation. Manchester: American Society for Gastrointestinal Endoscopy, 1994.

American Society for Gastrointestinal Endoscopy. *Antibiotic Prophylaxis for Gastrointestinal Endoscopy*. ASGE Publication 1027. Manchester: American Society for Gastrointestinal Endoscopy, 1995.

American Society for Gastrointestinal Endoscopy. *Sedation and Monitoring of Patients Undergoing Gastrointestinal Procedures*. ASGE Publication 1022. Manchester: American Society for Gastrointestinal Endoscopy, 1989 (revised 1995).

American Society for Gastrointestinal Endoscopy. *Risk Management. An Information Resource Manual*. Manchester: American Society for Gastrointestinal Endsocopy, 1990.

American Society for Gastrointestinal Endoscopy. *Appropriate Use of Gastrointestinal Endoscopy*. American Society for Gastrointestinal Endoscopy, revised November 2000.

Axon ATR, ed. *Infection in Endoscopy. Gastrointestinal Endoscopy Clinics of North America*, Vol. 3(3) (series ed. Sivak MV). Philadelphia: WB Saunders, 1993.

Bell GD. Premedication, preparation and surveillance. *Endoscopy* 2002; 34: 2–12.

British Society of Gastroenterology. Recommendations for standards of sedation and patient monitoring during gastrointestinal endoscopy. *Gut* 1991; 32: 823–7.

Cooper GS. *Indications and contraindications for upper gastrointestinal endoscopy*. In: *Gastrointestinal Endoscopy Clinics of North America* (series ed. Sivak MV). WB Saunders, 1994; 4(3): 439–54.

Cotton PB. Outcomes of endoscopic procedures: struggling towards definitions. *Gastrointest Endosc* 1994; 40: 514–18.

Cowen A. Infection and endoscopy: patient to patient transmission. In: Axon ATR, ed. *Infection in Endoscopy. Gastrointestinal Endoscopy Clinics of North America*, Vol. 3(3) (series ed. Sivak MV). Philadelphia: WB Saunders, 1993: 483–96.

Dajani AS, Bison AL, Chung KL *et al*. Prevention of bacterial endocarditis: recommendations by the American Heart Association. *J Am Med Assoc* 1990; 264: 2919.

Endocarditis Working Party of the British Society for Antimicrobial Chemotherapy. Antibiotic prophylaxis of infective endocarditis. *Lancet* 1990; 335: 88.

Fleischer DE. Better definition of endoscopic complications and other negative outcomes. *Gastrointest Endosc* 1994; 40: 511–14.

Freeman ML. *Sedation and monitoring for gastrointestinal endoscopy*. In: *Gastrointestinal Endoscopy Clinics of North America* (series ed. Sivak MV). WB Saunders 1994; 4(3): 475–99.

Meyer GW. Antibiotic prophylaxis for gastrointestinal procedures: who needs it? *Gastrointest Endosc* 1994; 40: 645–6.

Newcomer MK, Brazer SR. *Complications of upper gastrointestinal endoscopy and their management*. In: *Gastrointestinal Endoscopy Clinics of North America* (series ed. Sivak MV). WB Saunders 1994; 4(3): 551–70.

O'Connor HJ. Risk of sepsis in endoscopic procedures. In: Axon ATR, ed. *Infection in Endoscopy. Gastrointestinal Endoscopy Clinics of North America*, Vol. 3(3) (series ed. Sivak MV). Philadelphia: WB Saunders, 1993; 459–68.

Plumeri PA. *Informed consent for upper gastrointestinal endoscopy*. In: *Gastrointestinal Endoscopy Clinics of North America* (series ed. Sivak MV). Philadelphia: WB Saunders, 1994; 4(3): 455–61.

Quality safeguards for ambulatory gastrointestinal endoscopy. *Gastrointest Endosc* 1994; 40: 799–800.

Quality improvement of gastrointestinal endoscopy. *Gastrointest Endosc* 1993; 49: 842–44.

Quine MA, Bell GD, McCloy RF, Charlton JE, Devlin HB, Hopkins A. Prospective audit of upper gastrointestinal endoscopy in two regions of England; safety, staffing, and sedation methods. *Gut* 1995; 462–7.

Royal College of Anaesthetists. Implementing and ensuring safe sedation practice for healthcare procedures in adults. UK Academy of Medical Royal College and their faculties. Report of an Intercollegiate Working Party chaired by the Royal College of Anaesthetists. www.rcoa.ac.uk, 2002.

Rutala WA, Weber DJ. Creutzfeldt–Jakob disease: recommendations for disinfection and sterilization. *Clin Infect Dis* 2001; 32: 1348–56.

The recommended use of laboratory studies before endoscopic procedures. *Gastrointest Endosc* 1993; 39: 892–4.

The role of endoscopy in the management of esophagitis. *Gastrointest Endosc* 1988; 34(Suppl): 9S.

World Health Organization. *WHO infection control guidelines for transmissible spongiform encephalopathies*. WHO/CDS/CSR/APH/2000.3. Geneva:WHO, 1999.

ASGE Guidelines: Preparation for Endoscopy

Antibiotic prophylaxis for gastrointestinal endoscopy. *Gastrointest Endosc* 1995; 42: 630–5.

Guidelines on the management of anticoagulation and antiplatelet therapy for endoscopic procedures. *Gastrointest Endosc* 1998; 48: 672–5.

Monitoring equipment for endoscopy. *Gastrointest Endosc* 1995; 42: 615–7.

Practice guidelines for sedation and analgesia by non-anesthesiologists. *Anesthesiology* 1996; 84: 459–71.

Sedation and monitoring of patients undergoing gastrointestinal endoscopic procedures. *Gastrointest Endosc* 1995; 42: 626–9.

The recommended use of laboratory studies before endoscopic procedure. *Gastrointest Endosc* 1993; 39: 892–4.

Diagnostic Upper Endoscopy Techniques

4

Details of patient preparation are given in Chapter 3, along with some broad categories of indications. Clearly, both the endoscopist and the patient must be confident that the procedure is likely to be worthwhile and that it will be performed skillfully, with appropriate equipment and assistance.

PATIENT POSITION

The patient lies on the examination trolley/stretcher on the *left* side with the intravenous access line in the *right* arm. The height of the stretcher may be adjusted for comfort. The patient's head is supported on a small, firm pillow, so as to remain in a comfortable neutral position (Fig. 4.1). Monitoring devices are attached and supplemental oxygen may be given, usually via nasal prongs. Necessary sedation and/or pharyngeal anesthesia is applied. A biteguard is placed.

ENDOSCOPE HANDLING

The endoscopist should stand comfortably facing the patient, holding the instrument so that it runs in a gentle curve to the patient's mouth (Fig. 4.2).

The control head of the endoscope should be placed in the palm of the left hand, and held between the 4th and 5th fingers and the base of the thumb, with the tip of the thumb resting on the up/down control (Fig. 4.3). This grip leaves the 1st finger free to activate the air/water and suction buttons. The 2nd finger assists the thumb as a helper or 'ratchet' during major movements of the up/down control. With practice, the left/right control can be managed also with the left thumb (Fig. 4.4). Twisting the control body applies torque to the straightened shaft and is an important part of steering.

The right hand is used to push and pull the instrument, to apply torque rotation and to control accessories such as biopsy forceps.

PASSING THE ENDOSCOPE

Check that the patient is stable and comfortable and that the assisting nurse is ready. Select a standard forward-viewing endoscope and check it. Perform a white-light balance, lubricate the distal tip and double check the critical functions:

• tip angulation;

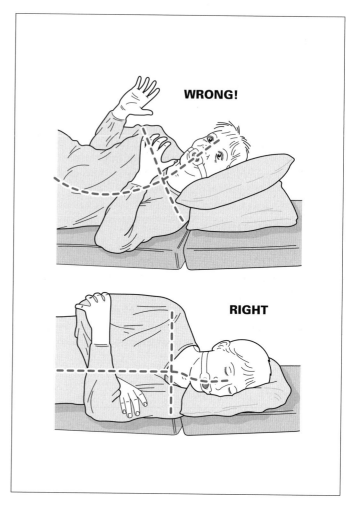

Fig. 4.1

- air and water;
- suction; and
- image quality.

Most endoscopists pass endoscopes under direct vision. Sometimes it may be necessary to insert the endoscope blindly, or with finger-guidance.

Check again that the patient is positioned easily for swallowing. The head should not be drooping, the neck slightly flexed, with the patient facing directly in front. After sedation, many patients slump into positions in which swallowing anything is a challenge.

Direct vision insertion

This is the best and standard method:

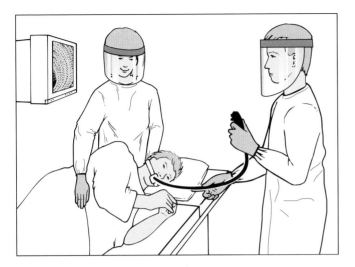

Fig. 4.2 A confident and balanced stance with a straight instrument, gently handled.

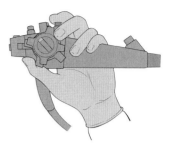

Fig. 4.3 The thumb rests on the up/down angulation control with the forefinger on the air/water valve; the middle finger can also assist.

- hold the endoscope head comfortably with the left hand, and the shaft with the right hand at the 30 cm mark.
- *rehearse up/down movements of the controls* to ensure that the tip will move in the correct longitudinal axis to follow the pharynx (Fig. 4.5). Adjust the lateral angulation control or twist the shaft appropriately so that the scope will travel down the midline.

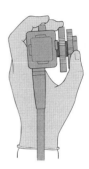

Fig. 4.4 The thumb can reach across to the left/right control.

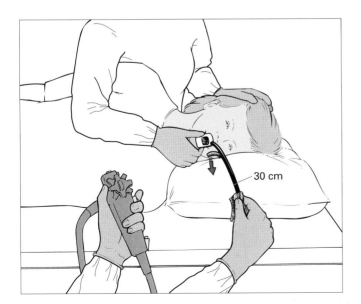

Fig. 4.5 The endoscopist pre-rehearses tip angulation in the correct axis before insertion.

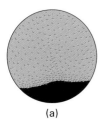

(a)

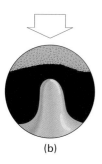

(b)

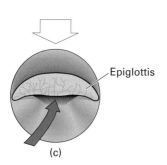

Epiglottis

(c)

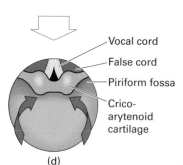

Vocal cord

False cord

Piriform fossa

Crico-
arytenoid
cartilage

(d)

Fig. 4.6 (a) Follow the centre of the tongue … (b) … past the uvula … (c) … and the epiglottis … (d) … to pass below the cricoarytenoid on either side.

• *pass the tip of the endoscope through the biteguard and over the tongue*, initially looking at the patient, not at the monitor.
• gently angle the tip 'up' (with your left thumb on the angulation control) as it passes over the tongue.
• *now look at the monitor.* Due to the looping of the endoscope, the view is inverted. Look for a rough, pale surface of the tongue horizontally in the upper (anterior) part of the view and keep the interface between it and the red surface of the palate in the centre of view by angling up appropriately, whilst advancing inwards over the curve of the tongue.
• *stay in the midline* by watching for the linear 'median raphe' of the tongue or the convexity of its midpart (Fig. 4.6a), correcting if necessary by twisting the shaft. The uvula is often seen transiently, projected *upwards* in the lower part of the view (Fig. 4.6b).
• *advance gently.* The epiglottis and, then, the cricoarytenoid cartilage with the 'false' vocal cords above it (and the vocal cords 2–3 cm beyond) are visible in the upper part of the view (Fig. 4.6c).
• the first, or pharyngeal, part of the esophagus is in tonic contraction and so is seen only transiently during swallowing. To reach it, angle downwards (posteriorly) so that the tip passes inferior to the curve of the cricoarytenoid cartilage, preferably passing to one or other side of the midline since the midline bulge of the cartilage against the cervical spine makes central passage difficult (Fig. 4.6d) and push inwards.
• *there is often a 'red-out'* as the tip impacts into the cricopharyngeal sphincter; insufflate air, maintain *gentle* inward pressure, ask the patient to swallow, and the instrument should slip into the esophagus within a few seconds. If necessary, ask the patient to swallow again, pushing gently as the sphincter opens.
• *keep watching carefully* to ensure smooth mucosal 'slide-by' as the instrument passes semi-blind into the upper esophagus, for this is where a diverticulum may occur.
    Throughout this process
• *be GENTLE*, feel the tube slide in
• coordinate gentle onward pressure with the patient's attempts to swallow
• *encourage the patient*, e.g. 'swallow, swallow again, well done … now take deep breaths'. This is best done by the endoscopist alone. Too many voices may confuse the patient, and suggest a degree of panic.
• if the view is lost, or a bulging tongue deflects the scope, or the teeth are seen, withdraw and start again.
• *be GENTLE*, force is dangerous and unnecessary.

Blind insertion

This technique (originating from the time when most gastroscopes were side-viewing, and still used for ERCP insertions) is a slight variation of the better direct vision method, but is done mainly by feel and by watching the patient, rather than looking at the endoscopic view on the monitor. The assistant maintains the patient's neck slightly flexed. With the right hand, the endoscopist passes the instrument tip through the mouthguard and over the tongue to the back of the mouth; using the left thumb on the control knob, the tip is then actively deflected upwards so that it curls in the midline over the back of the tongue and into the midline of the pharynx. The tip is advanced slightly and angled down a little, and the thumb is then removed from the tip control. Slight forward pressure is maintained, and the patient is asked to swallow as the 20 cm mark approaches the biteguard. There is an obvious feeling of 'give' as the tip passes the cricopharyngeal sphincter and then slides easily into the esophagus.

Finger-assisted insertion

This method is inelegant, and is needed only rarely, when standard methods fail. The control head of the instrument is held by an assistant (avoiding contact with the angulation controls). The biteguard is fitted over the shaft before insertion. The endoscopist puts the second and third fingers of the left hand over the back of the tongue. With the right hand, the tip of the instrument is passed over the tongue, and the inserted fingers of the left hand are used to guide it into the midline of the pharynx (Fig. 4.7). The fingers are withdrawn, the biteguard is slid into place, and the

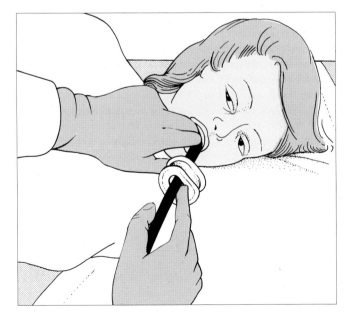

Fig. 4.7 Sometimes 'blind' insertion is helped by guiding the instrument between two fingers.

patient asked to swallow. If swallowing is not effective, the tip of the instrument has probably fallen into the left pyriform fossa.

Insertion with tubes in place

Endotracheal tubes present no problem for the endoscopist inserting under direct vision, the scope being angled down posterior to the tube and gently pushed through the sphincter. Deflating the cuff of the tube may be necessary occasionally to allow easier passage, especially with larger instruments. An existing naso-gastric tube may be a useful guide to the lumen. Withdrawing the endoscope may displace a naso-gastric or naso-enteric tube. This risk can be minimized by stiffening the tube with a guidewire.

ROUTINE DIAGNOSTIC SURVEY

Whatever the precise indication, it is usually appropriate to examine the entire esophagus, stomach and proximal duodenum, wherever possible. A complete survey may sometimes be prevented by stricturing from disease or previous surgery, or can be curtailed for other reasons.

It is important to develop a systematic routine to reduce the possibility of missing any area.

• the instrument is *always advanced under direct vision*, using air insufflation and suction as required, and delaying occasionally during active peristalsis (if antispasmotics have not been used).

• *mucosal views are often optimal during instrument withdrawal*, when the organs are fully distended with air, but inspection during insertion is also important since minor trauma by the instrument tip (or excessive suction) may produce small mucosal lesions with consequent diagnostic confusion.

• *lesions noted during insertion are best examined in detail* (and sampled for histology or cytology) following a complete routine survey of other areas.

• *as well as being systematic in survey, be precise in movements and decisive in making a 'mental map'* of what is being seen. A careful and complete examination can be achieved in less than 5–10 minutes by avoiding unnecessary movements and repeated examinations of the same area.

Golden rules for endoscopic safety:

• *do not push if you cannot see.*

• *if in doubt, inflate and pull back.*

Esophagus

There are several key landmarks in the esophagus:

• *the cricopharyngeal sphincter.*

• *indentation from the left main bronchus.*

- *pulsation of the left atrium and aorta.*
- *the esophagogastric (EG) mucosal junction* is clearly seen (at 38–40 cm from the incisor teeth in adults) where pale pink squamous esophageal mucosa abuts darker red gastric mucosa; this junction is often irregular and therefore called the 'Z-line'.
- *the diaphragmatic hiatus.* The diaphragm normally clasps the esophagus at or just below the EG junction. The position of the hiatus can be highlighted by asking the patient to sniff or to take deep breaths, and is recorded as the distance from the incisors. In any patient, the precise relationship of the Z-line to the diaphragmatic hiatus varies somewhat during an endoscopy (depending on the patient position, respiration, gastric distension, etc.). In normal patients, the gastric mucosa is often seen up to 1 cm above the diaphragm. An hiatus hernia is diagnosed if the Z-line remains more than 2 cm above the hiatus. From the clinical point of view, however, the presence or degree of herniation may be less important than any resulting esophageal lesions (e.g. esophagitis or columnar transformation).

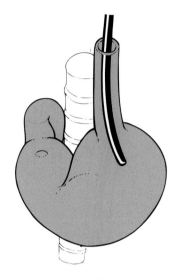

Fig. 4.8 The distal esophagus angles the scope into the posterior wall of the lesser curve.

Stomach

In the absence of stenosis, the endoscope can be advanced easily through the cardia and into the stomach under direct vision. The distal esophagus usually angles to the patient's left as it passes through the diaphragm, so it may be necessary to turn the instrument tip slightly to remain in the correct axis (Fig. 4.8). Unless the cardia is unduly lax, the mucosal view is lost momentarily as the tip passes through, passage being felt by the advancing hand as a slight 'give'. If the tip is further advanced in the same plane, it will abut on the posterior wall of the lesser curvature of the stomach so that pushing in blindly risks retroflexing towards the cardia. Thus,

- *rotate to the 'left' (anti-clockwise) to avoid the lesser curve,* and add air as the endoscope tip passes through the cardia.
- if there is no clear luminal view, withdraw slightly to disimpact the tip from the wall of the fundus or from the pool of gastric juice on the greater curve.

With the patient in the left lateral position and the instrument held correctly (buttons up), the disimpacted endoscopic view is predictable (Figs 4.9 & 4.10). The smooth lesser curvature is on the endoscopist's right with the angulus distally, the longitudinal folds of the greater curve are to the left and its posterior aspect is below:

- *aspirate any pool of gastric juice* to avoid reflux or aspiration during the procedure.
- *insufflate the stomach* enough to obtain a reasonable view during insertion.
- *inject a suspension of silicone* (simethicone) down the biopsy channel if there is excessive foaming.

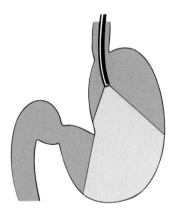

Fig. 4.9 With the gastroscope high on the lesser curve ...

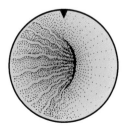

Fig. 4.10 ... the view is of the angulus in the distance, with the greater curve longitudinal folds a fluid pool on the left.

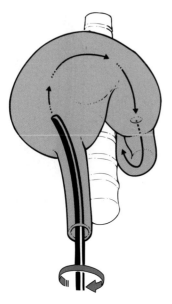

Fig. 4.11 The route to the pylorus and down the duodenum is a clockwise spiral around the vertebral column.

The four walls of the stomach are examined sequentially by a combination of tip deflection, instrument rotation and advance/withdrawal. The field of view during the advance of a four-way angling endoscope can be represented as a cylinder angulated over the vertebral bodies; the distended stomach takes up an exaggerated J-shape with the axis of the advancing instrument corkscrewing clockwise up and over the spine, following the greater curvature (Fig. 4.11). Thus, to advance through the stomach and into the antrum

- *angle the tip up increasingly;*
- *rotate the shaft clockwise.*

This clockwise corkscrew rotation through approximately 90° during insertion brings the angulus and antrum into end-on view (Fig. 4.12); it may be necessary now to deflect the tip a little downwards to bring it into the axis of the antrum (Fig. 4.13, 4.14), so that it runs smoothly along its greater curve. The motor activity of the antrum, pyloric canal and pyloric ring should be carefully observed. Asymmetry during a peristaltic wave is a useful indicator of present or previous disease.

Through the pylorus into the duodenum

The pyloric ring is approached directly for passage into the duodenum. During the maneuver it is convenient to use only the left

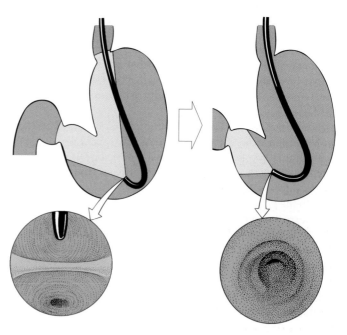

Fig. 4.12 The angulus and antrum come into view …

Fig. 4.13 … then angle down to see the pylorus in the axis of the antrum.

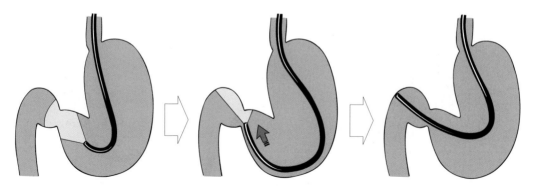

Fig. 4.14 The scope passes from the antrum …

Fig. 4.15 … to the pylorus and duodenal cap …

Fig. 4.16 … and tends to impact in the duodenum.

hand for tip angulation torque to maintain the instrument tip in the correct axis.

• *advance with the pyloric ring in the center of the view.* Passage is both felt and seen. Entry into the duodenal bulb is recognized by its granular and pale surface (Figs 4.15 & 4.16).

Patience may be needed to pass the pylorus, especially if there is spasm or deformity; *downward* angulation of the tip or deflation may help its passage. As the instrument tip passes the resistance of the pylorus, the loop which has inevitably developed in the stomach straightens out and accelerates the tip to the distal bulb (Fig. 4.16). So, to obtain optimal views of the duodenal bulb

• *withdraw a few cm to disimpact the tip* (and insufflate some air) to obtain a view (Fig. 4.17).

• *examine the bulb by circumferential manipulation of the tip* during advance and withdrawal. The area immediately beyond the pyloric ring, especially the inferior part of the bulb, may be missed by the inexperienced, who fail to withdraw sufficiently for fear of falling back into the stomach.

• *give an antispasmodic* (Buscopan® or glucagon) intravenously if visualization is impaired by duodenal motility.

• *avoid excessive air insufflation*, which will leave the patient uncomfortably distended.

Passage into the descending duodenum

The superior duodenal angle is the key landmark (Fig. 4.17) connecting the bulb and the descending duodenum. To pass into the descending duodenum, GENTLY

• advance so that the tip lies at the angle
• rotate the shaft about 90° to the right
• angle to the right
• angle up.

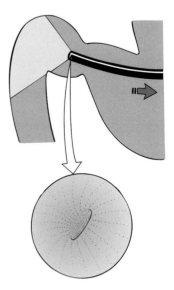

Fig. 4.17 Withdraw the scope to disimpact the tip and see the superior duodenal angle—an important landmark.

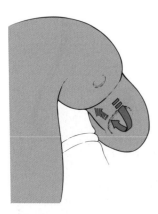

Fig. 4.18 Corkscrew the tip clockwise around the superior duodenal angle, using twist, right and up angulation simultaneously.

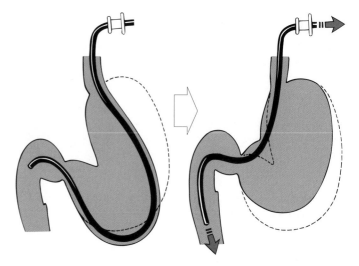

Fig. 4.19 Because of the loop in the greater curve …

Fig. 4.20 … withdrawal helps to advance the scope into the second part of the duodenum.

This maneuver effects a corkscrew motion around the angle (Fig. 4.18), and provides a tunnel view of the descending duodenum. Now, to advance further
- *do not simply push*, rather,
- *pull back*. Straightening the loop in the stomach propels the tip onwards, and the straightening shaft also corkscrews more efficiently round the superior duodenal angle (Figs 4.19 & 4.20). Using the correct 'pull and twist' method, the tip slides in to reach the ampullary region with only about 60 cm of instrument inserted. Duodenoscopy with more than 70 cm of shaft inserted is inelegant and uncomfortable.

A forward-viewing instrument gives tangential and often restricted views of the convex medial wall of the descending duodenum and the papilla of Vater. It may be possible to view this area with small calibre forward-viewing endoscopes in retroflexion (Fig. 4.21), but this is rarely necessary and not without risk. Much better views are obtained with side-viewing instruments.

Beyond the descending duodenum

Be gentle when trying to pass standard instruments into the third part of the duodenum and beyond. Pushing will initially only form a loop in the stomach (Fig. 4.22), and any further advance will come at the cost of considerable discomfort to the patient. It may be more effective (as with colonoscopy) to pull back, deflate, apply abdominal pressure, or change the patient's position. Deep duodenoscopy usually requires the use of specialized endoscopes.

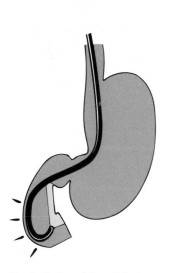

Fig. 4.21 Forceful partial retroflexion may give a view of the papilla, but take care.

Retroflexion in the stomach (J maneuver)

The fundus of the stomach is often best seen in retroversion, i.e. from below. To achieve this view safely:
• *place the tip of the endoscope in the mid stomach*, at or just beyond the angulus
• *insufflate air*
• *angle up acutely 180 degrees* (using both angulation controls). This maneuver should demonstrate the angulus, the entire lesser curve and the fundus as the instrument is withdrawn (Fig. 4.23)
• *pull back slowly and rotate the shaft* to obtain complete views of the fundus and cardia (Fig. 4.24)
• *do not pull back too far*. This risks impacting the retroverted tip in the distal esophagus!
• *after retroversion, remember to return the angulation controls to the neutral position.*

Retroversion in the stomach is probably best performed after examining the duodenum so as to avoid overinflation on the way in. Some patients (particularly those with a lax cardia) find it difficult to hold enough air to permit an adequate view. If retroversion proves difficult, it may be made easier by rotating the patient slightly onto the back to give the stomach more room to expand.

During all of these maneuvers, it is helpful to keep the shaft of the instrument relatively straight from the patient's teeth to your hands. This reduces the strain on the endoscope, helps orientation, and ensures that your rotating movements are precisely transmitted to the tip.

Removing the instrument

The mucosa should be surveyed carefully once again during withdrawal. Under the different motility conditions and organ shapes produced by distension and instrument position, areas previously seen only tangentially on insertion may be brought into direct view on the way out. The proximal lesser curve, a potential 'blind spot', merits particular attention as the scope withdraws along it. Remember to aspirate air (and fluid) from the stomach completely on withdrawal, and to release the brakes from the angulation controls (if they have been applied).

Finally, take a few seconds to reassure the patient, 'Well done, it's all over, we will talk in a few minutes …'.

Now begin the cleaning process!

It is important not to let blood and secretions dry on the instrument or in the channels. So, immediately
• *wipe the endoscope with a wet cloth*
• *place the tip in water and depress both control valves* (to flush out any mucus or blood form the air/water channel and wash through the instrumentation channel)

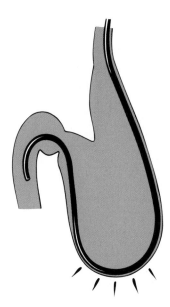

Fig. 4.22 Trying to reach the third part by force simply forms a loop in the stomach.

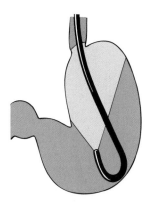

Fig. 4.23 Angulation of 180° retroflexes the tip to see the lesser curve …

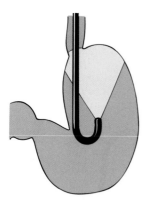

Fig. 4.24 … and swinging the retroflexed tip around gives a view of the fundus and cardia.

• *hand it over to the nurse/assistant* to enter the formal disinfection cycle.

PROBLEMS DURING ENDOSCOPY

Patient distress

Endoscopy should be terminated quickly if the patient shows distress of which the cause is not immediately obvious and remediable. Many patients have an understandable anxiety about choking. The airway should be checked and any residual oral secretions aspirated. If reassurance does not calm the patient, remove the instrument and consider giving additional sedation or analgesia (especially pethidine). Inadvertent bronchoscopy can occur if insertion is done by the 'blind' method and it is obvious from the unusual view and impressive coughing. Discomfort may arise from inappropriate pressure during intubation or from distension due to excessive air insufflation. Most sedated patients are able to belch; when performing endoscopy under general anesthesia it may be wise to keep the abdomen exposed so that overinflation can be detected, especially in children. Remember to keep inflation to a minimum and to aspirate all the air at the end of the procedure. Severe pain during endoscopy is very rare and indicates a complication such as perforation or a cardiac incident. It is extremely dangerous to ignore warning signs. Tachycardia and bradycardia may both indicate distress.

Getting lost

The endoscopist may become disorientated and the instrument looped in patients with congenital malrotations or major pathology (e.g. achalasia, large diverticula, hernias or ulcer scarring) or after complex surgery. Careful study of any available radiographs may help. The commonest reason for disorientation in patients with normal anatomy is inadequate air insufflation due to a defect in the instrument or air pump (which should have been detected before starting the examination). Inexperienced endoscopists often get lost in the fundus, especially when the stomach is angled acutely over the vertebral column. Having passed the cardia, the instrument tip should be deflected to the endoscopist's *left* and slightly downwards (Fig. 4.25). A wrong turn to the right will bring the tip back up into the fundus. When in doubt, withdraw, insufflate and turn sharply left to find the true lumen. A curious endoscopic view may indicate perforation (which is not always immediately painful). If in any doubt, abandon the examination and obtain radiological studies.

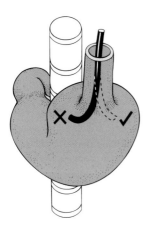

Fig. 4.25 Angling right (rather than left) on entering the fundus can cause retroflexion and can result in getting lost.

Inadequate mucosal view

Lack of a clear view means that the lens is lying against the mucosa or is obscured by fluid or food debris. Withdraw slightly and insufflate air; double check that the air pump is working and that all connections are firm with O-rings present. Try washing the lens with the normal finger-controlled water jet. This may not be effective if the instrument lens is covered by debris (or by mucosa which has been sucked onto the orifice of the biopsy channel). Pressure can be released by brief removal of the rubber valve of the biopsy port, but it may be necessary to flush the channel with water or air using a syringe. Small quantities of food or mucus obscuring an area of interest can be washed away with a jet of water. Foaming can be suppressed by adding a diluted emulsion of silicone (simethicone).

Since most patients comply with instructions to fast before procedures, the presence of excessive residue is an important sign of outlet obstruction. Standard endoscope channels are too small for aspiration of food; prolonged attempts simply result in blocked channels. The instrument can usually be guided along the lesser curvature over the top of the food to allow a search for a distal obstructing lesion. The greater curvature can also be examined if necessary by rotating the patient into the right lateral position. However, any examination in the presence of excess fluid or food carries a significant risk of regurgitation and pulmonary aspiration. The endoscopist should persist only if the immediate benefits are thought to justify the risk. It is usually wiser to stop and to repeat the examination only after proper gastric lavage.

RECOGNITION OF LESIONS

This book is concerned mainly with techniques, rather than with lesions. The accompanying CD-ROM contains some illustrations of lesions which may be encountered. We recommend also that beginners should study several of the excellent atlases that are now available. Certain points, however, are worth emphasizing here.

Esophagus

Esophagitis normally follows acid reflux and is most apparent distally, close to the mucosal junction. There is no clear macroscopic dividing line from normality; the earliest visible changes consist of mucosal congestion and edema which obscure the normal fine vascular pattern. At a more advanced stage the mucosa becomes friable and bleeds easily on touching; there are patches of exudate and areas of reddening or ulceration, usually in the long axis of the esophagus. The process culminates in a symmetrical stricture above which the mucosa (now protected from reflux) may appear almost normal. Columnar lining of the esophagus (Barrett's esophagus) is easily recognized. Red gastric-type mucosa extends more than 2 cm above the diaphragmatic hiatus; initially in longitudinal stripes or plaques, it can coalesce to involve the entire circumference. Monilial esophagitis is characterized by white spots or plaques.

Esophageal carcinoma usually causes asymmetrical stenosis, with areas of exuberant abnormal mucosa and sometimes an irregular ulcer with raised edges. Carcinoma of the gastric fundus may also infiltrate upwards submucosally to involve the esophagus. The correct diagnosis is then easily made if the endoscope can be passed through the stricture to allow retroverted views of the cardia.

Diverticula in the mid- or distal esophagus are easily recognized, but the instrument may enter a pulsion diverticulum (Zenker's) or pouch in the upper esophagus without the true lumen being seen at all. Lack of view and resistance to inward movement are (as always) an indication to pull back and reassess. Webs or rings, such as the Schatzki ring, at or just proximal to the esophagogastric junction may not be obvious to the endoscopist due to a combination of 'flat' bright endoscope illumination and distortion from the wide-angled lens view. If in doubt, skilled radiology (with video taping) should be used to define the situation before therapeutic endoscopy.

Varices lie in the long axis of the esophagus as tortuous bluish mounds covered with relatively normal mucosa. They resemble varicose veins elsewhere in the body.

Mallory–Weiss tears are 5–20 mm longitudinal mucosal splits lying either side of or across the esophagogastric mucosal junction. In the acute phase the tear is covered with exudate or clot and may sometimes be seen best in a retroverted view.

Motility disturbances of the esophagus should be diagnosed by radiology and manometry, but their consequences—such as dilation, pseudodiverticula, food retention and esophagitis—are well seen at endoscopy, which is always needed to rule out obstructing pathology. Hypermotility is probable when recurrent esophageal contractions are seen in spite of antispasmodics and sedation; the incoordinate non-propulsive contractions of esophageal dysfunction being known as 'tertiary' contractions.

Achalasia allows the endoscope to pass easily through the cardia, in contrast to the fixed narrowing of pathological strictures due to reflux esophagitis or malignancy.

Stomach

The appearance of the normal gastric mucosa varies considerably. Reddening (hyperaemia) may be generalized (e.g. with bile reflux into the operated stomach) or localized; sometimes it occurs in long streaks along the ridges of mucosal folds. Localized (traumatic) reddening with or without petechiae or edematous changes is often seen on the posterior upper lesser curve in patients who habitually retch. Macroscopic congestion does not correlate well with underlying histological gastritis, and care should be taken when considering clinical relevance. Biopsy samples should be taken when any abnormality is suspected, and tests for *Helicobacter pylori* performed in patients with dyspepsia with or without macroscopic lesions (see p. 55).

Gastric folds vary in size but the endoscopic assessment also depends upon the degree of gastric distension. Very prominent fleshy folds are seen in Ménétrier disease and are best diagnosed by a snare loop biopsy. Patients with duodenal ulceration often have large gastric folds with spotty areas of congestion within the areae gastricae and excess quantities of clear resting juice. With gastric atrophy, there are no mucosal folds (when the stomach is distended) and blood vessels are easily seen through the pale atrophic mucosa. Atrophy is often associated with intestinal metaplasia, which appears as small, gray-white plaques.

Erosions and ulcers are the most common localized gastric lesions. A lesion is usually called an erosion if it is small (<5 mm diameter) and shallow, with no sign of scarring. Acute ulcers and erosions are often seen in the antrum and may be capped with, and partially obscured by, clots. Edematous erosions appear as small, smooth, umbilicated raised areas, often in chains along the folds of the gastric body. When these are multiple the condition has been called 'chronic erosive gastritis'. However, gastritis is a term best reserved for histological use.

The classic chronic benign gastric ulcer is usually single and is most frequently seen on the lesser curvature at or above the angulus. It is typically symmetrical with smooth margins and a clean base (unless eroding adjacent structures). Multiple and punched out ulcers (sometimes oddly shaped and very large) occur in some patients taking non-steroidal anti-inflammatory drugs (NSAIDs).

Malignancy may be suspected if an ulcer has raised irregular margins (or different heights around the circumference), a lumpy hemorrhagic base or a mucosal abnormality surrounding the ulcer. Mucosal folds around a benign ulcer usually radiate towards it and reach the margin. Inexperienced endoscopists cannot hope to separate benign from malignant ulcers on macroscopic appearance alone; tissue specimens must always be taken. Unfortunately, gastric cancer is usually diagnosed at an advanced stage in Western countries, when it is all too obvious at endoscopy. Diffusely infiltrating carcinoma (*linitis plastica*) may be missed unless motility is carefully studied. Early gastric cancer may mimic a small benign ulcer, chronic erosion or a flat polyp. Polypoid lesions under 1 cm in diameter are usually inflammatory in origin. However, since all malignant lesions start small and are curable if detected at an early stage, odd mucosal lumps and bumps should never be ignored; a tissue diagnosis must be made. Submucosal tumors are characterized by normal overlying mucosa and bridging folds; leiomyomas and plaques of aberrant pancreatic tissue (characteristically found in the floor of the antrum) usually have a central dimple or crater.

Duodenum

Duodenal ulcers, either current or previous, often cause persistent deformity of the pyloric ring. The ulcers occur most commonly on the anterior and posterior walls of the bulb and are frequently multiple. When active they are surrounded by edema and acute congestion. Scarring often results in a characteristic shelf-like deformity which partially divides the bulb and may produce a pseudodiverticulum; a small linear ulcer or scar is seen running along the apex of this fold. The mucosa of the bulb often reveals small mucosal changes of dubious clinical significance. Areas of mucosal congestion with spotty white exudate ('pepper and salt' ulceration) merge into even less definite macroscopic appearances labelled as 'duodenitis'. Small mucosal lumps in the proximal duodenum usually reflect underlying Brunner gland hyperplasia or gastric metaplasia (ectopic islands of gastric mucosa). Duodenal tumors occur mainly in the region of the papilla of Vater.

Ulceration and duodenitis in the second part of the duodenum suggests Zollinger–Ellison syndrome or underlying pancreatic disease. Crohn's disease may be suspected by the presence of small aphthous ulcers in the second part; typical granulomas may be seen on histology.

Celiac disease can be recognized macroscopically (in the second part of the duodenum and beyond), especially when viewed close up. The fine villus pattern is lost and the mucosa appears knobbly and edematous.

Dye enhancement techniques

Dye enhancement techniques may assist the recognition of inconspicuous mucosal lesions such as those found in celiac disease. Dye spraying (chromoscopy) is best achieved by spraying with a tube and fine nozzle applied close to the mucosa. The dye fills the interstices, highlighting irregularities in architecture. Indigo carmine is used most frequently but simple pen ink (1 : 5 dilution of washable blue) is also effective. Intravital staining is an alternative approach to lesion enhancement. Stains such as methylene blue, Lugol solution and toluidine blue may be taken up preferentially in diseased mucosa (such as intestinal metaplasia). Fluorescent stains (given intravenously) may highlight lesions under special conditions such as ultraviolet illumination.

SPECIMEN COLLECTION

It is important to emphasize the need for close collaboration between endoscopy and laboratory staff. The diagnostic yield from endoscopic specimens will be maximized if laboratory staff are involved in defining the methods for specimen handling and transmission. Specimens should reach the laboratory with precise details of their origin and the specific clinical question that needs to be answered. Pathologists who routinely receive a copy of the endoscopy findings (and later follow-up) are more likely to give timely and relevant reports. Regular review sessions should be part of the quality improvement process.

Biopsy techniques

Biopsy specimens are taken with cupped forceps. The lesion should be approached face-on, so that firm and direct pressure can be applied to it with the widely opened cups. Pressure is easier to apply if the forceps are kept close to the endoscope tip. Better control is achieved by advancing the scope to the target rather than the forceps. Similarly, specimens from the esophagus are best taken by angling the tip of the endoscope acutely against the wall with the forceps barely protruding. The forceps are closed gently but firmly by an assistant and withdrawn. At least six good specimens should be taken from any lesion—perfectionists would ask for many more. Forceps with a central spike make it easier to take specimens from lesions that have to be approached tangentially (e.g. in the esophagus). Some experts prefer not to use spiked forceps because of the risk of accidental skin puncture.

Ulcer biopsies should include samples from the base and from the ulcer rim in all four quadrants; basal specimens are sometimes diagnostic but usually yield only slough. When sampling proliferative tumors it is wise to take several specimens from the same place to penetrate the outer necrotic layer. A larger final tumor biopsy may be obtained by grabbing a protuberant area and deliberately *not* pulling the forceps through the channel; the instrument is withdrawn with the specimen still outside the tip.

The methods for handling and fixing specimens should be established after discussion with the relevant pathologist; some prefer samples to be gently flattened on paper or other surfaces such as cellulose filter (Millipore etc.). The cellulose filter method of biopsy mounting has considerable advantages for the management of multiple small endoscopic biopsies. They adhere well to the filter and are rarely lost; they are mounted in sequence so that errors of location are impossible; and they allow the histopathologist to view serial sections of six to eight biopsies at a time in a row across a single microscope slide. A 15 mm strip of cellulose filter (just less than the width of a glass slide) has a pencil-ruled or printed central line and a notch or mark made at one end (Fig. 4.26a). Each biopsy is eased out of the forceps cup with the tip of a micropipette or toothpick (to avoid needle-stick injuries) (Fig. 4.26b), placed exactly onto the line and patted flat (Fig. 4.26c). The strip with its line of biopsies is placed into fixative (Fig. 4.26d). In the laboratory it is processed, wax-mounted in the correct orientation (Fig. 4.26e), sectioned through the line of biopsies on the filter (Fig. 4.26f), positioned on the microscope slide (Fig. 4.26g), and then stained and examined without handling the biopsies individually at any stage. A dissecting microscope or hand lens can be used to orientate mucosal specimens before fixation if information is required about the mucosal architecture (e.g. duodenal biopsies in malabsorption).

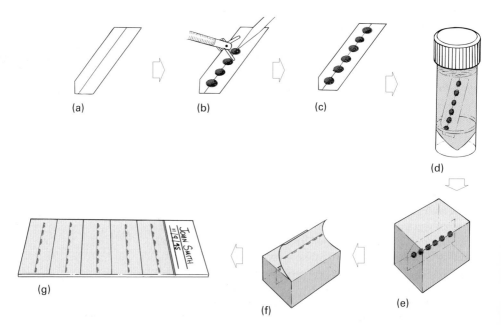

Fig. 4.26 Stages in placing biopsies onto the filter then fixing, sectioning and mounting the specimens.

Detection of *Helicobacter pylori* infection is important. A biopsy specimen should be taken from the gastric antrum (if on PPIs also from body and fundus) and placed in a rapid urease test; a formalin-fixed specimen may be taken to be sent to the laboratory if the urease test is negative.

Biopsy sites often bleed trivially but sometimes sufficiently to obscure the lesion before adequate samples have been taken; if so, the area should be washed with a jet of water or a 1:100 000 solution of epinephrine (adrenaline). Bleeding of clinical significance is exceptionally rare.

Cytology techniques

Cytology specimens are taken under direct vision with a sleeved brush (Fig. 4.27) which is passed through the instrument channel. The head of the brush is advanced out of its sleeve and rubbed and rolled repeatedly across the surface of the lesion; a circumferential sweep of the margin and base of an ulcer is desirable. The brush is then pulled back into the sleeve and both are withdrawn together. The brush is protruded, wiped over two to three glass slides and then rapidly fixed before drying damages the cells. The precise method of preparation (in the unit or laboratory) should be determined by the cytologist. Brushes should not be re-used. Bleeding of clinical significance is exceptionally rare. A trap (Fig. 4.28) can be used to collect cytology specimens. Suction through the channel after a biopsy procedure ('salvage cytology') also produces useful cellular material.

The value of brush cytology depends largely on the skill and enthusiasm of the cytopathologist. Many studies indicate that a combination of brush cytology and biopsy provides a higher yield than biopsy alone. In practice most endoscopists reserve cytology for lesions from which good biopsy specimens are difficult to obtain (e.g. tight esophageal strictures) and for resampling a suspicious lesion. Taking aspiration samples for cytology though a needle may occasionally be useful.

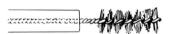

Fig. 4.27 Cytology brush with outer sleeve.

Sampling submucosal lesions

Standard biopsy specimens are usually normal in patients with submucosal lesions (such as benign tumors), since the forceps do not traverse the muscularis mucosae. Larger and deeper specimens can be taken with a diathermy snare loop; the technique is described with polypectomy in Chapter 7. Larger specimens can also be taken with 'jumbo' forceps or even larger experimental forceps which have to be 'muzzle loaded', i.e. the forceps are threaded backwards up the biopsy channel before the instrument is passed into the patient, using an overtube (Fig. 4.29) to protect the pharynx and esophagus during intubation. An alternative method for obtaining deeper tissue samples is

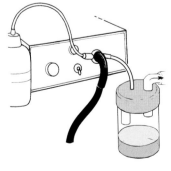

Fig. 4.28 A suction trap to collect fluid specimens.

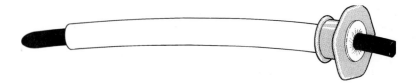

Fig. 4.29 An overtube with biteguard over a rubber lavage tube.

to use a needle to obtain aspiration samples for cytology. Good results have been reported for this technique but it has not become popular.

DIAGNOSTIC ENDOSCOPY UNDER SPECIAL CIRCUMSTANCES

Operated patients

Unless prevented by postoperative stenosis, endoscopy is the best method for diagnosis and exclusion of mucosal inflammation, recurrent ulcers and tumors after upper GI surgery. The endoscopist can document the size and arrangement of any outlet or anastomosis, but barium radiology and nuclear medicine techniques may be needed to give more information about motility and emptying disorders.

Experience is needed to appreciate the wide range of 'normal' endoscopic appearance in the operated patient. Partial gastrectomy, gastroenterostomy and pyloroplasty result in reflux of bile and intestinal juice; resultant foaming in the stomach may obscure the endoscopic view and should be suppressed by flushing with a silicone suspension. Gastric distension is difficult to maintain in patients with a large gastric outlet; avoid pumping too much air and overdistending the intestine. Most patients who have undergone partial gastrectomy or gastroenterostomy have impressively hyperemic mucosae. Initially this is most marked close to the stoma, but atrophic gastritis is progressive and plaques of grayish white intestinal metaplasia may be seen. There is an increased risk of cancer in the gastric remnant, particularly close to the stoma. Many cancers in this site are not recognized endoscopically, so during endoscopy of an operated stomach the opportunity should be taken to obtain multiple biopsy (and cytology) specimens from within 3 cm of the stoma—in every case, whatever the level of suspicion.

Ulcers following partial gastrectomy or gastroenterostomy usually occur at or just beyond the anastomosis. Endoscopic diagnosis is usually simple, but the area just beneath the stoma may sometimes be difficult to survey completely using a forward-viewing instrument. A lateral-viewing endoscope may also sometimes allow a more complete survey in a scarred and tortuous pyloroplasty. Many surgeons use non-absorbable sutures when performing an intestinal anastomosis; these can ulcerate through the mucosa and appear as black or green threads and loops. Their clinical significance remains controversial; when sutures are associated with ulcers, it is justifiable to attempt their removal with biopsy forceps or with a diathermy snare loop. Endoscopy is occasionally performed (for bleeding or stomal obstruction) within a few days of upper GI tract surgery; if so, air insufflation should be kept to a minimum.

Acute upper gastrointestinal bleeding

Bleeding provides special challenges for the endoscopist and details are given in Chapter 5.

Endoscopy in children

Pediatric endoscopy is relatively simple with appropriate instruments and preparation; examination techniques are similar to those used in adults. The standard adult forward- and lateral-viewing instruments (8–11 mm diameter) can be used down to the age of about two years. Smaller pediatric instruments (5 mm diameter) may be needed in infants.

Endoscopy can be performed with little or no sedation in the first year of life. Fasted babies usually swallow the instrument avidly. Many endoscopists prefer to use general anesthesia beyond this age and into the mid-teens (especially for complex procedures) but some are satisfied with conscious sedation alone. This usually consists of a small dose of a benzodiazepine and generous doses of pethidine (Demerol). Even an apparently calm or well-sedated child may suddenly become briefly uncontrollable during intubation and it is essential to swaddle the upper body and arms completely within a blanket before beginning, and to have an experienced nurse in charge of the biteguard (and suction). There is a risk of excessive air insufflation when using heavy sedation or anesthesia; it is wise to keep the abdomen exposed during examination and to palpate it regularly. Careful monitoring of oxygenation and the pulse is essential. Impending shock in a neonate is indicated by the baby suddenly becoming still and floppy; this is an indication to abort the procedure rapidly.

FURTHER READING

Blades EW, Chak A, eds. *Upper Gastrointestinal Endoscopy.* In: *Gastrointestinal Endoscopy Clinics of North America*, Vol. 4(3) (series ed. Sivak MV). Philadelphia: WB Saunders, 1994.

Jaffe PE. *Technique of upper gastrointestinal endoscopy.* In: *Gastrointestinal Endoscopy Clinics of North America* (series ed. Sivak MV). Philadelphia: WB Saunders, 1994; 4(3): 501–21.

Gilbert DA, Marino AJ, Jensen DM *et al.* Hot biopsy forceps. *Gastrointest Endosc* 1992; 38: 753–6.

Koop H. Gastroesophageal reflux disease and Barrett's esophagus. *Endoscopy* 2002; 34(2): 97–103.

Lambert R. Diagnosis of esophagogastric tumors. *Endoscopy* 2002; 34: 129–38.

MacKenzie J. Push enteroscopy. *Gastrointest Endosc Clin North Am* 1999; 9: 29–36.

Pediatric Gastrointestinal Endoscopy (guest editor VL Fox). In: *Gastrointestinal Endoscopy Clinics of North America* (series ed. Sivak MV). Philadelphia: WB Saunders, 2001.

Sampliner RE. Practice guidelines on the diagnosis, surveillance, and therapy of Barrett's esophagus. The Practice Parameters Committee of the American College of Gastroenterology. *Am J Gastroenterol* 1998; 93: 1028–32.

The role of endoscopy in the surveillance of premalignant conditions of the upper gastrointestinal tract. *Gastrointest Endosc* 1998; 48: 663–8.

VanDam J, ed. *The Oesophagus.* In: *Gastrointestinal Endoscopy Clinics of North America,* Vol. 4(4) (series ed. Sivak MV). Philadelphia: WB Saunders, 1994.

Wu JCY, Sung JJY. Ulcer and gastritis. *Endoscopy* 2002; 34: 104–10.

Therapeutic Upper Endoscopy

Gastroenterologists now have a major role in the interventional treatment of many upper gastrointestinal problems. Established techniques include the management of dysphagia (due to benign and malignant esophageal stenoses and achalasia), polyps, gastric and duodenal stenoses, foreign bodies, acute bleeding and nutritional support. Other exciting therapies, for example the endoscopic treatment of reflux, and of obesity, are being developed.

BENIGN ESOPHAGEAL STRICTURES

Gastro-esophageal reflux is the commonest cause of benign esophageal strictures. Other causes include specific esophageal inflammations and infections, medications, caustic ingestion, radiation, extrinsic compression, and therapeutic interventions (surgery, endoscopy and radiation).

In general, dysphagia occurs when the esophageal lumen is less than about 13 mm. It follows that easy passage of a standard endoscope (8–10 mm diameter) does not exclude a problem, or the possible need for treatment.

Dilation methods

Dilation is used only as part of an overall treatment plan, with due attention also to diet, lifestyle modification, and necessary medications. Surgery is needed in a few recalcitrant cases.

There are many dilation techniques and varieties of equipment.

Mild strictures can be treated simply in some patients with mercury-weighted dilators (such as Maloney bougies) without sedation. Dilating balloons or graduated bougies are used when the stenosis is tight or tortuous, under endoscopic and/or fluoroscopic control (over a guidewire), to ensure correct placement. Both methods are effective and their relative merits are debated. Bougie techniques give a better 'feel' of the stricture, which may be an important safety factor.

Certain strictures, particularly those due to irradiation or corrosive ingestion, are more difficult to dilate. Procedures may need to be repeated several times with gradual increase in dilator size—too rapid an increase can result in perforation.

Dilation can provoke bacteremia, so antibiotic prophylaxis against endocarditis should be given to patients with significant cardiac lesions (see Table 3.1).

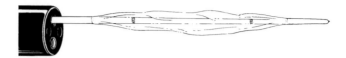

Fig. 5.1 A deflated 'through-the-scope' (TTS) balloon dilator and guide-wire.

Balloon dilation

Balloons are designed to be passed through the endoscope channel, often with a guide-wire (Fig. 5.1). They range from 3 to 8 cm in length and from 10 to 15 mm in diameter. Most strictures are short, but medium-length balloons (about 5 cm) are convenient to use since they are less likely to 'pop out' of the stricture than shorter ones. Lubrication should be applied, either directly to the balloon with a silicone spray or by injecting 1–2 mL of silicone oil down the endoscope channel followed by 10 mL of air. The stricture is examined endoscopically, and its diameter assessed. Tight strictures should be approached initially with small balloons. The guide-wire and soft tip of an appropriately sized balloon is passed gently through the stricture under direct vision. The balloons are fairly translucent, so that it is usually possible to observe the 'waist' endoscopically during the procedure and to judge the effect. Balloons are distended with water (or contrast medium) to the pressure recommended by the manufacturer conventionally for 2 minutes.

The 'through-the-scope' (TTS) balloon dilation technique has several advantages. It can be performed as part of the initial endoscopy, and does not normally require fluoroscopic monitoring. The results should be obvious immediately, and the endoscope can be passed through the stricture to complete the endoscopic examination.

Bougie dilation

This is performed with graduated bougies that are passed over a guidewire. This ensures that the dilator will pass correctly through the stricture (and not into a diverticulum or necrotic tumor, or through the wall of a hiatus hernia). This security exists only if the position of the wire is checked frequently, using fluoroscopy or a fixed external landmark. Fluoroscopic monitoring is essential when tight and complex strictures are being treated.

Savary–Guilliard bougies are popular. These are simple tapering plastic wands with radio-opaque markers (Fig. 5.2). Variants of this design are available from other manufacturers. Diameters range from 3 to 20 mm.

The following steps should be performed when dilating:
• *place the guidewire through the endoscope* into the gastric antrum.

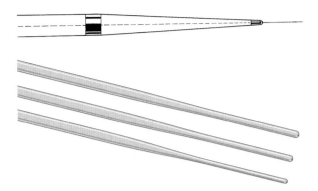

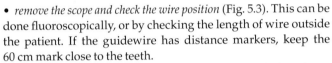

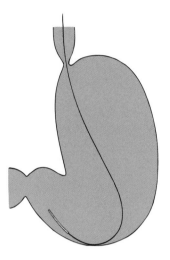

Fig. 5.2 Tips of Savary–Guilliard (above) and American Endoscopy (below) dilators for use over a guidewire.

Fig. 5.3 A dilator guidewire positioned in the gastric antrum.

- *remove the scope and check the wire position* (Fig. 5.3). This can be done fluoroscopically, or by checking the length of wire outside the patient. If the guidewire has distance markers, keep the 60 cm mark close to the teeth.
- *choose a bougie that will pass relatively easily through the stricture* and slide it over the guidewire down close to the mouth; lubricate the tip of the bougie.
- *hold the bougie shaft in the left hand and push in,* simultaneously applying counter-traction on the guidewire with the right hand. Keep the left elbow extended so that the dilator cannot travel too far when resistance 'gives' (Fig. 5.4). This reduces the chance of advancing too rapidly.
- *increase the size of the bougies progressively,* checking the guidewire position repeatedly, but *observe the rule of three,* i.e. do not use more than three sizes above the size at which significant resistance is first felt.
- *after dilation, check the effect endoscopically.* Take biopsy and cytology samples if necessary.

Post-dilation management

Patients should be kept nil by mouth and under observation for at least 1 h after dilation. Any complaint of pain should be taken seriously. Chest films and a water-soluble contrast swallow should be performed if there is any suspicion of perforation (perforation is discussed in detail under 'Esophageal cancer palliation' below). A trial drink of water is given if progress has been satisfactory. The patient is then discharged with instructions to keep to a soft diet overnight, plus appropriate medications and a follow-up plan. Dilation can be repeated within a few days in severe cases, and then subsequently every few weeks until swallowing has been restored fully.

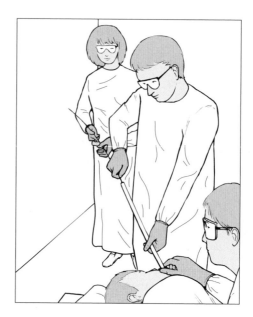

Fig. 5.4 Advance the dilator with the left hand and the elbow extended to avoid sudden overinsertion. Keep traction on the wire with the right hand.

ACHALASIA

Manometry provides the gold standard for the diagnosis of achalasia, but endoscopy is also essential to exclude submucosal or fundal malignancy. Achalasia can be treated with surgical or laparoscopic myotomy, balloon dilation, or with injections of botulinum toxin.

Balloon dilation

Patients with achalasia often have food residue in the esophagus. They should take only a clear liquid diet for several days before the procedure, and large-bore tube lavage may be needed beforehand.

Many different techniques and balloons have been used. The balloon position can be checked radiologically, or under direct vision with the endoscope alongside the balloon shaft (Fig. 5.5), or even by a retroversion maneuver with the balloon fitted over the endoscope shaft. We prefer to place a guidewire endoscopically, identify the lower esophageal sphincter fluoroscopically, and then dilate with a balloon under fluoroscopic control.

Achalasia balloons are available with diameters of 30, 35 and 40 mm. It is wise to start with the smallest balloon, warning the patient that repeat treatments may be necessary if symptoms persist or recur quickly.

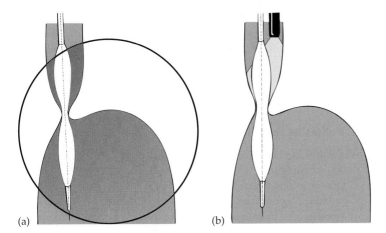

Fig. 5.5 Achalasia dilating balloons (before full inflation). (a) Checked fluoroscopically. (b) Visualized endoscopically.

Inflation is maintained at the recommended pressure for up to one minute, and may be repeated. Observe the waist on the balloon fluoroscopically: inadequate expansion may indicate other pathology. Conversely, abrupt disappearance of the waist may suggest perforation (perforation is discussed under 'Esophageal cancer palliation' below).

There is usually some blood on the balloon after the procedure. Close observation is mandatory for at least 4 h. Chest radiographs and a water-soluble contrast swallow are done routinely in some units. Nothing should be given by mouth until the patient and the radiographs have been examined by the endoscopist personally. A trial drink of water is given under supervision. The uncomplicated patient can return to a normal diet on the next day.

Botulinum toxin

Treatment with botulinum toxin can be applied by direct free-hand endoscopic injection into the area of the lower esophageal sphincter, or using endoscopic ultrasound guidance. Results are good, but short-lived, so that the value of this method is still not clear.

ESOPHAGEAL CANCER PALLIATION

Barium studies and endoscopy have complementary roles in assessing the site and nature of esophageal neoplasms. Endoscopic ultrasonography is the most accurate staging tool. Endoscopic management can help to improve swallowing in the majority of patients who are unsuitable for surgery because of intercurrent disease or tumor extent. However, endoscopists should be aware of their treatment limitations, and balance technological enthusiasm with full consideration of the patient's quality of life (and likely duration of survival). Even achieving a large lumen will not restore normal swallowing. The goal should be to achieve adequate swallowing, at the lowest risk and inconvenience to the patient.

Palliative techniques

Several methods can be used to palliate malignant dysphagia. The abrupt onset of severe dysphagia may be due to the impaction of a food bolus, which can be removed endoscopically by standard techniques. Malignant strictures can be dilated using wire-guided balloons or bougies, taking great care not to split the tumor by being overambitious. The bulk of an exophytic tumor can be reduced by various ablation techniques. Monopolar diathermy is readily available, but it is difficult to control the depth of injury, and charring occurs quickly. Local injection of a toxic agent like absolute alcohol is also effective, if somewhat unpredictable. Laser ablation (using the Nd:YAG laser) was popular in previous years, largely because a 'no-touch' technique seemed esthetically preferable, but the equipment is expensive, and similar results can be achieved using APC (argon plasma coagulation), which is simpler and cheaper. It also has the advantage that the energy can be applied tangentially.

Ablative techniques are most useful in short exophytic lesions, and for recurrences after surgery or stenting. All of the methods are somewhat hazardous (perforation rate up to 5%) and are rarely effective for more than a few weeks. As a result, there is an increasing tendency to place stents as a primary measure. Chemotherapy, radiotherapy and photodynamic therapy are also used.

Esophageal stenting

There are good indications for using esophageal stents, but insertion can be very challenging, and is not to be undertaken lightly, by the endoscopist or patient.

The best candidates are mid-esophageal tumors in patients with a prognosis limited to weeks or months, and in those with tracheo-esophageal fistulae. Stents cannot be used when the tumor extends to within 2 cm of the cricopharyngeus. Stents may function less well in lesions at the cardia because of the angulation, and reflux may be a problem. Great care must be taken when dysphagia is caused by very large tumors, since stent placement may compromise the airway. Prior bronchoscopy is appropriate in such cases, and trial inflation of a balloon may indicate what diameter is tolerable.

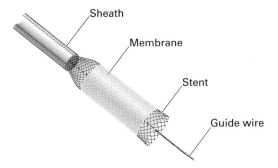

Sheath

Membrane

Stent

Guide wire

Fig. 5.6 Covered metal mesh stent.

Stent variety

Plastic stents have largely been replaced with expandable metal mesh stents, since they are easier and less hazardous to insert. Many types are now available. They vary by the type, diameter and weave of the wires (which determine their expansile strength), by their shapes and sizes, and by the presence or absence of a covering membrane (Fig. 5.6). This membrane is helpful in patients with fistulae, and reduces tumor ingrowth, but some mesh must left exposed to prevent migration. Stents for use in the esophagus have luminal diameters of 15–24 mm, and lengths of 6–15 cm. They are compressed into delivery systems of 6–11 mm. Most expand gradually over a few days, and become fully incorporated in the esophageal wall so that they cannot be removed. Less powerful stents—although easy to place and well tolerated—may not expand sufficiently to relieve the patient's symptoms, even with balloon dilation.

Stent insertion

The patient is fully informed about the aims, the potential serious risks of the procedure, and the (few) alternatives. Antibiotic prophylaxis should be considered. The lesion is assessed carefully by radiology and endoscopy, and bougie dilation is performed if necessary (to about 12 mm), to allow passage of the endoscope if possible. The upper and lower margins of the tumor are marked by endoscopic injection of contrast medium, using a sclerotherapy needle. A guidewire is placed, and its position checked by fluoroscopy.

The stent system is then introduced over the guidewire and the stent is released by gradual withdrawal of the sleeve. Correct positioning of the stent is judged fluoroscopically (using the contrast medium marks), and then by repeat endoscopy.

Post-stent management

Patients are usually kept in the hospital overnight under observation, because of the immediate risk of perforation and bleeding, and for necessary pain control. Chest and water-soluble contrast swallow radiographic studies are performed after about 2 hours. Clear fluids can be given after 4 hours if there have been no adverse developments.

Patients must understand the limitations of the stent, and the need to maintain a soft diet with plenty of fluids during and after meals. Written instruction should be provided and relatives counseled. Overambitious eating or inadequate chewing may result in obstruction. If food impaction occurs, the bolus can usually be removed or fragmented endoscopically using snares, biopsy forceps or balloons.

Stent dysfunction due to tumor overgrowth can be managed by endoscopic ablation or placement of another stent inside the first. Gastro-esophageal reflux can be a problem with stents crossing the cardia. Patients may need to sleep propped up, and to use acid-reducing medications. Occasionally, a good result from chemotherapy or radiotherapy may make it possible to remove a stent. For the same reason, stents (especially the covered variety) may migrate spontaneously. Recovery of stents from the stomach can be challenging.

Esophageal perforation

The endoscopic treatment of esophageal strictures is relatively safe in most cases using optimal techniques. However, perforations do occur, especially with complex and malignant strictures approached by inexperienced or overconfident endoscopists. The rate is approximately 0.1% in benign esophageal strictures, 1% in achalasia dilation, and 5–10% in treatment of malignant lesions. The risk is minimized by taking the process step by step—gradually and deliberately. Never try to dilate to the largest balloon or bougie simply because it is available.

Early suspicion and recognition of perforation is the key to successful management, and no complaint should be ignored. The problem is usually obvious clinically; the patient is distressed and in pain. Signs of subcutaneous emphysema may develop within a few hours. Radiographic studies should be performed. Surgical consultation is mandatory when perforation is seriously suspected or confirmed. Many confined perforations have been managed conservatively, with nil oral intake, intravenous fluids and antibiotics—with or without placement of a sump tube across the perforation. The choice between surgical and conservative management (and the timing of surgical intervention if conservative management appears to be failing) is often difficult; review of the literature shows varied and strong opinions.

Conservative management is more likely to be appropriate when the perforation is in the neck; because the mediastinum is not contaminated, local surgical drainage can be performed simply when necessary. Perforation through a tumor can be treated immediately with a covered stent, if the lumen can be found, and if surgical cure is not possible.

GASTRIC AND DUODENAL STENOSES

Functionally significant stenoses may occur in the stomach or duodenum as a result of disease (tumors and ulcers) and following surgical intervention (e.g. hiatus hernia repair, gastroenterostomy, pyloroplasty and gastroplasty). Balloon dilation of stenosed surgical stomas is usually effective (except in the case of banded gastroplasty with a rigid silicone ring). Pyloroduodenal stenosis caused by ulceration can be relieved by balloon dilation, but recurrence is common. Expandable stents are being used with remarkably good effect in patients with malignant stenosis of the stomach and duodenum.

GASTRIC AND DUODENAL POLYPS AND TUMORS

Endoscopic polypectomy is used very frequently in the colon, and many of the techniques (see Chapter 7) can be applied in the stomach and duodenum. Polyps are much less common in the stomach and duodenum than in the colon, and are rare in the esophagus. Many of these polyps are sessile, and some are largely submucosal, making endoscopic treatment more difficult and hazardous. The possibility of a transmural lesion should be considered, and endoscopic ultrasonography may be helpful in making a treatment decision; surgical (or laparoscopic) resection may be safer. Injecting the base of sessile gastric and duodenal polyps with epinephrine (adrenaline; 1 : 10 000) may make removal easier, and may reduce the risk of bleeding. Some endoscopists use detachable loops for the same purpose.

Endoscopic mucosal resection (EMR) has been developed in Japan for removal of sessile lesions up to 2 cm or more in diameter. The lesion is raised up by injecting a cushion of saline/epinephrine, and then sucked into a special transparent plastic cap attached to the tip of the endoscope. The lesion is then resected with a snare loop incorporated in the cap (Fig. 5.7, see also Fig. 7.43).

Snare diathermy techniques can be used also to obtain large biopsy specimens when the gastric mucosa appears thickened, and when standard biopsy techniques have failed to provide a diagnosis.

Gastric polypectomy, EMR and snare-loop biopsy techniques can cause bleeding and perforation. They also leave an ulcer; it is wise to prescribe acid-suppressant medication for a few weeks.

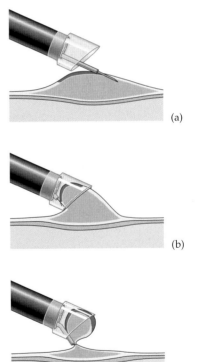

(a)

(b)

(c)

Fig. 5.7 Endoscopic mucosal resection. (a) Inject a saline cushion below the lesion. (b) Suck the lesion into the transparent cap. (c) Snare and resect the lesion.

FOREIGN BODIES

Foreign bodies are mainly a problem in children, in elderly patients with poor teeth, and in the drunk or deranged. The problem is obvious if the patient suddenly cannot swallow, and especially if a missing object is visible on a radiograph. However, many instances are less straightforward. Patients may not know that they have swallowed a foreign object. Some common items (e.g. bones and drink-can tags) are not radio-opaque. It is therefore necessary to maintain a high index of suspicion.

Chest and abdominal radiographs (with lateral views) are appropriate. A water-soluble contrast swallow examination is helpful in some patients, but it is not necessary, and is potentially hazardous if dysphagia is complete.

Many foreign bodies pass spontaneously, but active treatment should be initiated within hours in some circumstances.

Urgent treatment is required for:
- *patients who cannot swallow saliva*;
- *impacted sharp objects*;
- *ingestion of button batteries* (which can disintegrate and cause local damage).

Foreign body extraction

Objects impacted at or above the cricopharyngeus are usually best removed by surgeons with rigid instruments. Flexible endoscopy now takes precedence in most (but not all) other situations. The use of an overtube increases the therapeutic options (Fig. 5.8). Endoscopy can usually be accomplished with conscious sedation, but general anesthesia should be considered in children and uncooperative adults, and when there is concern about the airway.

Food impaction

An intravenous injection of glucagon (0.5–1.0 mg) may help release a food impaction. The use of meat tenderizer is discouraged, since severe pulmonary complications have resulted. Meat can be removed as a single piece endoscopically, using a polypectomy snare, triprong grasper or retrieval basket. Another approach is to use strong suction on the end of an over-

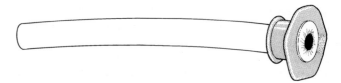

Fig. 5.8 An overtube with biteguard.

tube or a banding sleeve. Take care not to lose the bolus near the larynx. Food that has been impacted for several hours can usually be broken up (e.g. with a snare), and the pieces pushed into the stomach. This must be done carefully, especially if there is any question of a bone being present. Sometimes it is possible to maneuver a small endoscope past the food bolus and to use the tip to dilate the distal stricture; the food can then be pushed through the narrowed area.

Most patients with impacted food have some esophageal narrowing (due to a benign reflux stricture or Schatski's ring). The endoscopist's task is not complete until this has been checked and treated. Usually, dilation can be performed at the time of food extraction, but should be delayed if there is substantial edema or ulceration.

Gastric bezoars

Gastric bezoars are aggregations of fibrous animal or vegetable material. They are usually found in association with delayed gastric emptying (e.g. postoperative stenosis or dysfunction). Most masses can be fragmented with biopsy forceps or a polypectomy snare, but more distal bolus obstruction may result if fragmentation is inadequate. Various enzyme preparations have been recommended to facilitate disruption, but these are rarely necessary or effective. Large gastric bezoars are best disrupted and removed by inserting a large-bore lavage tube, and instilling and removing 2–3 L of tap water with a large syringe. The cause of gastric-emptying dysfunction should be evaluated, and treated.

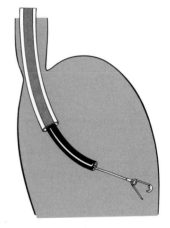

Foreign bodies

The range of swallowed objects is amazing. Foreign bodies trapped in the esophagus should always be removed. Sharp objects (such as open safety pins) are best withdrawn into the tip of an overtube (Fig. 5.9); sometimes it is safer to use a rigid esophagoscope.

Most objects that reach the stomach will pass spontaneously, but there are exceptions, which demand early intervention.

Indications for early removal of foreign bodies

• Sharp and pointed objects have a 15–20% chance of causing perforation (usually at the ileo-cecal valve), and should be extracted while still in the stomach or proximal duodenum.
• Objects > 2 cm diameter and longer than 5 cm are unlikely to pass from the stomach spontaneously and should be removed if possible.

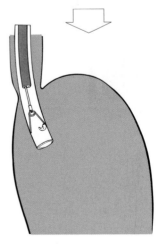

Fig. 5.9 Remove sharp foreign bodies with a protecting overtube.

Button batteries usually pass spontaneously when they have reached the stomach; a purgative should be given to accelerate the process.

Foreign bodies rarely pass out of the stomach in children who have had pyloromyotomies.

Endoscopists should resist the temptation to attempt removal of condoms containing cocaine or other hard drugs since rupture can lead to a massive overdose; surgical removal is the safest option.

Golden rules for foreign body removal

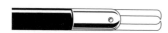

Fig. 5.10 Foreign-body extraction forceps.

- *Be sure that your extraction procedure is really necessary.*
- *Think before you start, and rehearse outside the patient.*
- *Do not make the situation worse.*
- *Do not be slow to get surgical or anesthesia assistance.*
- *Protect the esophagus, pharynx and bronchial tree during withdrawal (with an overtube or endotracheal anesthesia).*
- *Remove sharp objects with the point trailing.*

Extraction devices

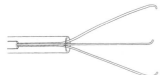

Fig. 5.11 A triprong grasping device.

The endoscopist should have several specialized tools available, in addition to the overtube. There are forceps with claws or flat blades designed to grasp coins (Fig. 5.10); a triprong extractor is useful for meat (Fig. 5.11). Many objects can be grasped with a polypectomy snare or stone-retrieval basket. Others can be collected in a retrieval net. Any object with a hole (such as a key or ring) can be removed by passing a thread through the hole. The endoscope is passed into the stomach with biopsy forceps or a snare closed within its tip, grasping a thread which passes down the outside of the instrument (Fig. 5.12). The forceps are advanced and the thread passed through the object, dropped and retrieved from the other side.

ACUTE BLEEDING

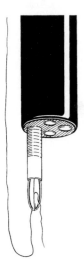

Fig. 5.12 Take a thread down with the forceps to pass through any object with a hole in it, such as a ring or key.

Acute upper GI bleeding (hematemesis and/or melena) is a common medical problem, for which endoscopy has become the primary diagnostic and therapeutic technique. Emergency endoscopy is a challenging task. There is considerable potential for benefit, but also for risk. These techniques require experience, nerve and judgment. Safety considerations are paramount. The endoscopist should be well trained, working with familiar equipment and expert nurses. Unstable patients should be under supervision in an intensive care environment. Sedation should be given cautiously, and precautions taken to avoid pulmonary aspiration. Patients with severe bleeding are often best examined under general anesthesia, with the airway protected by a cuffed endotracheal tube.

Many different endoscopic techniques have been developed. These include injection with saline/epinephrine or sclerosant or fibrin, banding, thermal probes (heat probe, bipolar or monopolar electrocoagulation, APC and lasers) and clipping. Endoscopic suturing will soon be added to this list. Many trials have compared different techniques, but the experience of the endoscopist—and familiarity with a particular technique—is probably the most important determinant of success. Laser photocoagulation initially became popular because it was assumed that it was safer not to touch the lesion. However, it has become clear that direct pressure with some probes (and injection treatment) provides an important tamponade and 'coaptation' effect (see Fig. 5.18), and increases the size of vessel that can be treated.

The *timing* of endoscopy is important. Examination can be delayed to a convenient time (e.g. the next morning) in patients who appear to be stable, but the endoscopic team must be prepared to go into action within hours (after immediate resuscitation) in certain circumstances.

Indications for emergency endoscopy

- *Continued active bleeding requiring intervention.*
- *Suspicion of variceal bleeding.*
- *Presence of an aortic graft.*
- *Severe rectal bleeding with inconclusive colonic studies.*
- *Elderly patients with cardiovascular compromise on presentation.*

Lavage?

Blood clots may obscure the view in the stomach and duodenum. Standard gastric lavage is rarely effective, even when performed personally with a large-bore tube. Endoscopes with a large channel (or two channels) allow better flushing and suction. An alternative approach is to start the procedure with an overtube over the endoscope (Fig. 5.13). If blood is encountered, the endoscope can be removed, and blood clots sucked directly through the overtube; lavage can be performed.

A diagnosis can usually be made even if the stomach cannot be emptied completely. Lesions are rare on the greater curvature, where the blood pools in the standard left lateral position.

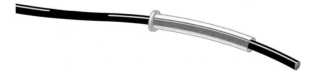

Fig. 5.13 Overtube with endoscope.

Changing the patient's position somewhat should improve the survey, but turning completely on the right side is hazardous unless the airway is protected.

Bleeding lesions

Lesions that cause acute bleeding are well known. Endoscopy has highlighted the fact that many patients are found to have more than one mucosal lesion (e.g. esophageal varices and acute gastric erosions). Thus, a complete examination of the esophagus, stomach and duodenum should be performed in every bleeding patient, no matter what is seen en route. A lesion should be incriminated as the bleeding source only if it is actively bleeding at the time of endoscopy, or shows characteristic stigmata (see p. 74), for example, an ulcer with adherent clot or a visible vessel. If the patient has presented with hematemesis, and complete upper endoscopy shows only a single lesion (even without any of these features), it is likely to be the bleeding source. This is not necessarily the case if the presentation has been with melena, or if the examination takes place more than 48 hours after bleeding, since acute lesions such as mucosal tears and erosions may already have healed. Likewise, varices cannot be incriminated definitely unless they are bleeding or show specific stigmata.

Variceal treatments

Endoscopic treatment of esophageal (and gastric) varices can be helpful in patients who are bleeding, or who have recently bled. Prophylactic treatment remains controversial. Intervention in the presence of active bleeding is challenging. Patients are often very sick, and the views may be poor. It may be helpful to tilt the patient slightly head up, or to apply traction on a gastric balloon to reduce the flow of blood. Often it is wise to defer endoscopy for several hours, pending the effect of pharmacological treatment. Sengstaten–Blakemore tube tamponade or TIPS (Transjugular Intrahepatic Portosystemic Shunt) treatments may be appropriate.

Elimination of varices usually involves a series of treatments. Endoscopic management should be seen as only part of a patient's overall care.

Available techniques include injection sclerosis, banding and combination techniques. Clips and loops have also been used recently.

Injection sclerotherapy

Injection sclerotherapy has been used for decades. Many adjuvant devices have been described, including overtubes with a lateral window and the use of balloons—either in the stomach to compress distal varices or on the scope itself to permit tamponade if bleeding occurs. However, most experts use a simple 'free-hand' method, with a standard large-channel endoscope and a flexible, retractable needle (Fig. 5.14). Injections are given directly into the varices, starting close to the cardia (and below any bleeding site) and working spirally upwards for about 5 cm. Each injection consists of 1–2 mL of sclerosant, to a total of 20–40 mL.

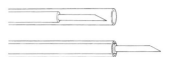

Fig. 5.14 A retractable sclerotherapy needle.

Precise placement of the needle within the varix (as guided by co-injection of a dye such as methylene blue or by simultaneous manometric or radiographic techniques) may improve the results and reduce the complications. However, some experts believe that paravariceal injections are also effective, and it is often difficult to tell which has been achieved. If bleeding occurs on removal of the needle, it is usually helpful to tamponade the area simply by passing the endoscope into the stomach. The esophago-gastric junction can be compressed directly if the endoscope is retroflexed.

Sclerosants

Several chemical agents are available as sclerosants. Sodium morrhuate (5%) and sodium tetradecylsulfate (STD) (1–1.5%) are popular in the USA. Polidocanol (1%), ethanolamine oleate (5%) and STD are widely used in Europe. Efficacy, ulcerogenicity and the risk of complications run together, since it is the process of damage and healing by fibrosis that eradicates or buries the communicating veins, but may also cause stricturing. Endoscopic polymer injection is another alternative. The two cyanoacrylate agents most commonly used are not available in the USA. These polymers solidify almost immediately on contact with aqueous material. The endoscopist and nurse must use them carefully to provide an effective injection without gluing up the endoscope. Results are excellent, especially in gastric varices (which do not respond well to standard sclerotherapy). Many use this technique also in patients who relapse quickly after banding or sclerotherapy in the acute situation. Other 'glues' are being evaluated.

Variceal banding

This has become popular because it causes fewer ulcers and strictures than sclerotherapy. The device consists of a friction-fit sleeve on the endoscope tip, an inner cylinder preloaded with elastic bands and a trip wire that passes up the endoscope channel (Fig. 5.15). The varix is sucked into the sleeve, and the band released by pulling on the wire. Multiple bands are applied in an upwards spiral fashion every 1–2 cm. Banding can be applied also to gastric varices and to small ulcers (e.g. Dieulafoy lesions).

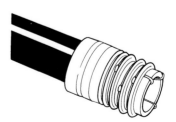

Fig. 5.15 An esophageal banding device.

Care after variceal treatments

The risks of variceal treatment include all of the complications of emergency endoscopy (especially pulmonary aspiration).

Patients often have transient chest pain, odynophagia (pain on swallowing) and dysphagia. They should maintain a soft diet for a few days, avoid any medications that may irritate or cause bleeding, and take acid-suppressing agents. Treatment should be repeated in about a week in the context of acute bleeding, but should be delayed for several weeks when elective, to allow the lesions to heal. Delayed complications include esophageal stricturing, which is more common after sclerotherapy. Strictures can be dilated gingerly with standard methods.

Treatment of bleeding ulcers

Duodenal and gastric ulcers are still common causes of acute bleeding. About 80% will stop bleeding spontaneously. It is important if possible to predict those patients likely to rebleed and select them for endoscopic treatment. We are guided by the size of the initial bleed, the overall status of the patient, and by the presence or absence of stigmata.

Ulcer stigmata

The following stigmata provide useful pointers when considering treatment options.
- *Active 'spurters' continue to bleed (or rebleed soon) in 70–80% of cases.*
- *Ulcers with a 'visible vessel' have about a 50% chance of rebleeding.*
- *Clean ulcers do not rebleed.*

An important question is whether it is appropriate to wash clots off the base of an ulcer simply to check for these stigmata. Most endoscopists will do so in high-risk patients provided they are poised for treatment.

Treatment modalities

The most popular hemostatic methods currently are injection, heat probe, bipolar probe and combinations. Clips are being used increasingly.

Injection treatment. Epinephrine in saline (1 : 10 000) is applied with a sclerotherapy needle in 0.5–1.0 mL aliquots around the base of the bleeding site, up to a total of 10 mL. Some prefer to use absolute alcohol in much smaller volumes (1–2 mL in 0.1 mL aliquots) or combinations of epinephrine with alcohol, or with the sclerosants used for the treatment of varices.

The *heat probe* (Fig. 5.16) provides a constant temperature of 250°C. First tamponade, then apply several pulses of 30 J.

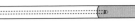

The *bipolar (or multipolar) probe* (Fig. 5.17) provides bipolar electrocoagulation, which is assumed to be safer than monopolar diathermy (which produces an unpredictable depth of damage). Use the larger 10 French gauge probe at 30–40 W for 10 seconds.

Fig. 5.16 Teflon-coated tip of a heat probe with a water-jet opening.

These treatment devices share some common principles. All can be applied tangentially, but (apart from injection) are better used face-on if possible. When the vessel is actively bleeding, direct probe pressure on the vessel or feeding vessel will reduce the flow and increase the effectiveness of treatment (Fig. 5.18). The bipolar and heat probes incorporate a flushing water jet, which helps to prevent sticking.

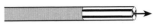

Fig. 5.17 The tip of a multipolar probe with a central water jet.

Clipping (Fig. 5.19). Metal clips can be applied endoscopically, and are particularly useful for small bleeding ulcers (e.g. Dieulafoy lesions), for Mallory–Weiss tears, and large visible vessels.

Know when to stop treatment! Treatment attempts should not be protracted if major difficulties are encountered; the risks rise as time passes. There are some patients and lesions in which endoscopic intervention may be foolhardy, and surgery is more appropriate, for example, a large posterior wall duodenal ulcer that may involve the gastroduodenal artery. Angiographic treatment is useful in selected cases.

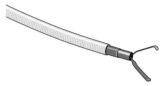

Fig. 5.19 Hemostatic clip.

Follow-through after treatment. A single endoscopic treatment is not an all-or-nothing event. It is necessary to continue other medical measures, to maintain close monitoring and to plan ahead for further intervention (pharmacological, endoscopic, radiological or surgical) if bleeding continues or recurs. The job is not complete until the lesion is fully healed. Eradication of *Helicobacter pylori* should reduce the risk of late rebleeding.

Treatment of bleeding vascular lesions

All of the endoscopic methods can be used to treat vascular malformations such as angiomas and telangiectasia. The risk of full-thickness damage and perforation is greater in organs

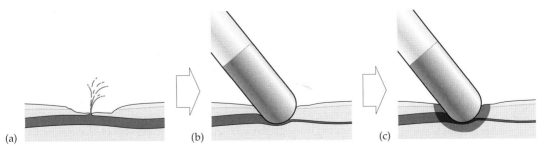

(a)   (b)   (c)

Fig. 5.18 (a) Bleeding ulcer. (b) Probe pressure stops the blood flow and coapts the vessel wall. (c) Coagulation.

with thinner walls (e.g. the esophagus and duodenum) than in the stomach. Lesions with a diameter of more than 1 cm should be approached with caution, and treated from the periphery inwards to avoid provoking hemorrhage. Bipolar and heat probe, and the argon plasma coagulator provide the best control.

Complications of hemostasis

The most important hazards of endoscopic hemostasis are pulmonary aspiration and provocation of further bleeding. It is difficult to know how often endoscopy causes rebleeding that would not have occurred spontaneously, but major immediate bleeding is unusual and can usually be stopped. The risk of pulmonary aspiration is minimized by protecting the airway using pharyngeal suction and a head-down position, or a cuffed endotracheal tube. Perforation can be caused by any of the treatment methods if they are used too aggressively, especially in acute ulcers, which have little protecting fibrosis.

ENTERAL NUTRITION

There are several ways in which endoscopists can assist patients who need nutritional help. Temporary support can be provided by placement of a nasoenteric feeding tube. Permanent nutritional support requires the creation of a gastrostomy (or jejunostomy).

Feeding and decompression tubes

Tubes for short-term feeding (and gastric decompression) are normally placed blindly at the bedside, but can also be passed under fluoroscopic guidance or after endoscopic placement of a guidewire. Two direct endoscopic methods can be used when necessary, for example to advance tubes through the pylorus or a surgical stoma.

Through-the-channel method

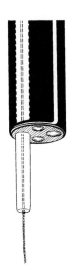

Fig. 5.20 The feeding tube and guidewire are passed through a large-channel scope.

The simplest technique is to advance a 7–8 French gauge plastic tube through a large-channel endoscope, over a standard (400 cm long) 0.035-inch diameter guidewire (Fig. 5.20). The tube and guidewire are advanced through the pylorus under direct vision, and subsequent passage is checked by fluoroscopy. When the tip is in the correct position, the endoscope is withdrawn whilst further advancing the tube (and guidewire) through it. Finally, the guidewire is removed and the tube is rerouted through the nose. Another method is to pass a guidewire through the biopsy channel into position in the small bowel. The endoscope is then removed and a feeding tube is fed over the guidewire into position.

Alongside-the-scope method

This technique allows the placement of a tube larger than the endoscope channel. The feeding tube is stiffened with one or more guidewires. A short length of suture material is attached to the end of the tube and is grasped within the instrument channel with a snare (Fig. 5.21). The endoscope is passed into the stomach and close to the pylorus. The snare and tube are then guided through the pylorus (or stoma) under direct vision. Once in position (checked by fluoroscopy), the thread is released and the endoscope is removed. The proximal end of the tube is rerouted from the mouth to the nose. The final position is checked by fluoroscopy, withdrawing any excess loops in the stomach.

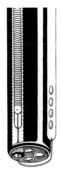

Fig. 5.21 A tube is carried alongside the scope by a thread grasped with a snare or forceps.

A variant of this method has proven useful recently. The feeding tube (again stiffened with one or more guidewires) is passed through the nose and into the stomach. The endoscope is passed through the mouth, and is used to push the tip of the tube through the pylorus. The endoscope is then passed alongside the tube into the duodenum. The tube advances by the friction between the scope and the tube. The tube is held firmly at the nose, and the scope is withdrawn to the pylorus and then advanced again to push the tube deeper.

Percutaneous endoscopic gastrostomy (PEG)

Nasoenteric feeding can be used for several weeks but is inconvenient and unstable, and it is probably often responsible for pulmonary aspiration and pneumonia. PEG is now a popular method for long-term feeding, and may permit the transfer of patients with chronic neurological disability from acute care hospitals into nursing homes. The PEG technique can be extended into a feeding jejunostomy by the use of appropriate tubes.

Studies comparing PEG with operative gastrostomy have shown some advantages for the endoscopic method, but surgical (and laparoscopic) options should always be considered, especially in circumstances where the endoscopic approach may be more difficult or hazardous (e.g. after gastric surgery).

Antibiotics are usually given to reduce the risk of skin sepsis.

There are two main methods for PEG placement—the 'pull' and the 'push' methods.

The 'pull' technique

This, the original method, is still the most commonly used.
1 A standard endoscope is passed into the stomach and the gastric outlet is checked.

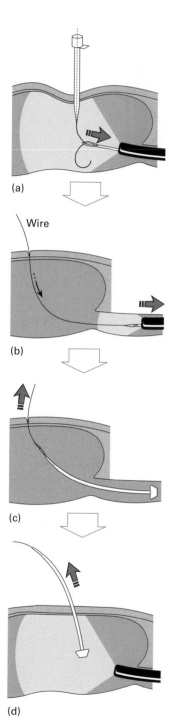

(a)

Wire

(b)

(c)

(d)

Fig. 5.22 PEG. (a) Grasp the wire. (b) Pull the wire through the mouth. (c) Pull the PEG tube down the esophagus. (d) Pull bumper to gastric wall.

2 The patient is rotated onto the back, the stomach distended with air and the room darkened (this is particularly important when using videoscopes).

3 The tip of the endoscope is directed towards the anterior wall of the stomach.

4 The abdominal wall is observed for transillumination and the assistant indents the site with a finger.

5 The endoscopist checks that the indentation can be seen in an appropriate part of the body of the stomach.

6 The assistant marks this spot on the anterior abdominal wall, applies disinfectant and infiltrates local anesthetic into the skin, subcutaneous tissues and fascia.

7 A short (5–10 mm) skin incision is made with a pointed blade, extending into the subcutaneous fat.

8 The assistant pushes an 18 gauge needle catheter (loaded onto a syringe half-full of water) through the anterior abdominal wall, aspirating after initial penetration. Air should not bubble back until the needle is visible endoscopically (showing that it is in the stomach, not in another organ such as the colon). The endoscopist places a snare in front of the area of indentation, and needle entry, and maintains gastric distension. A wire at least 150 cm long with loops at both ends is passed through the needle and grasped with the snare (Fig. 5.22a).

9 The endoscope and snare are withdrawn through the mouth (Fig. 5.22b), carrying the wire loop, ensuring that the external end of the wire remains outside of the abdominal wall.

10 The wire loop coming out of the mouth is then attached to the PEG tube, which is pulled down the esophagus (Fig. 5.22c), and through the anterior abdominal wall (Fig. 5.22d). The tube should not be pulled tight, to avoid compression necrosis of the gastric wall. Leave about 1 cm of 'play', as judged endoscopically.

11 The tube is shortened and then anchored at the skin with one of various disk devices.

12 Feeding can start on the day after the procedure (with a trial of water initially) if there are no complications.

13 The patient and all relevant care-givers are given detailed instructions on tube care, and what to do if problems arise.

14 The initial tube can usually be replaced by a flat feeding button after about 2 months.

The 'push' technique

This follows steps 1 through 8 above, to the point where the needle catheter is in the stomach, with the endoscope poised in front of it. A long straight guidewire is then pushed through the needle, and grasped endoscopically with a snare. The scope and snare are removed via the mouth, so that there is a long wire extending from the mouth through the stomach and through the abdominal wall. Keeping tension on both ends of the wire, a special PEG tube is then slid all the way over the wire. The tip of the tube is grasped as it exits the abdominal wall, and pulled into place. An external bolster is attached.

Direct introducer technique

This is used in some countries, especially by radiologists. The feeding tube is pushed through the abdominal wall, rather than pulling it down from the mouth. The stomach is distended with air using a nasogastric tube under fluoroscopy. A needle catheter, trochar and straight guidewire are passed through the abdominal wall into the stomach. A succession of dilators are passed over the wire, and eventually a PEG tube collapsed in a sleeve. The sleeve is removed and the PEG withdrawn into position. This method eliminates contamination of the PEG tube by passage through the mouth, but it is difficult to choose the correct puncture position unless endoscopy is used. It is sometimes also difficult to push the trochar and catheter through the abdominal and stomach walls.

PEG problems and risks

PEG placement cannot be performed in patients with esophageal strictures that are too tight to permit the passage of an endoscope. Technical difficulties and risks are higher in patients who have previously undergone abdominal surgery, particularly with partial gastric resection, and in patients with gastric varices, marked ascites or obesity.

Specific risks of PEG

There are three main types of risk.
• *Perforation/fistula.* Avoid injuring other organs (such as the colon) by making sure that good transillumination is achieved, and by using the bubble-back check. A small pneumoperitoneum is not uncommon, and is usually benign, but major and persisting leakage requires operative correction.
• *Local infection* can occur (even necrotizing fasciitis), particularly if the skin incision is too small or if the tube has been pulled too tight against the gastric wall (one of the most common errors). Pre-procedure antibiotics reduce this risk.
• *Tube dislodgement* can result in peritonitis and may require surgical repair. Dislodgement after 10–14 days usually leaves a track (for 12–24 hours) during which the tube can be replaced (carefully).

Percutaneous endoscopic jejunostomy (PEJ)

Jejunal feeding is often recommended to reduce the risk of pulmonary aspiration, especially in patients with gastro-esophageal reflux and gastroparesis. The jejunostomy tube may be inserted (under endoscopic guidance) through an established PEG tract or using special commercial kits at the time of the original PEG puncture. Placing a jejunostomy tube directly into the small bowel, by analogous transillumination/puncture techniques, is currently under investigation.

Nutritional support

The purpose of these endoscopic interventions is to provide safe and effective nutritional support. It is thus important to ensure that the patient and all involved caregivers are instructed appropriately about tube care and feeding regimens. They also need structured follow-up support.

FURTHER READING

Allum WH, Griffin SM, Watson A, Colin-Jones D on behalf of the Association of upper gastrointestinal surgeons of Great Britain and Ireland, The British Society of Gastroenterology, and the British Association of Surgical Oncology. Guidelines for the management of oesophageal and gastric cancer. *Gut* 2002; 50(Suppl V): v1–23.

American Society for Gastrointestinal Endoscopy. *Guideline for Management of Ingested Foreign Bodies.* ASGE Publication 1026. American Society for Gastrointestinal Endoscopy, 1995.

American Society for Gastrointestinal Endoscopy. Role of PEG/PEJ in enteral feeding. *Gastrointest Endosc* 1998; 48: 699–701.

American Society for Gastrointestinal Endoscopy. Stents for gastrointestinal strictures. *Gastrointest Endosc* 1998; 47: 588–93.

American Society for Gastrointestinal Endoscopy. The role of endoscopic therapy in the management of variceal hemorrhage. *Gastrointest Endosc* 1998; 48: 697–8.

Bhasin DK, Malhi NJS. Variceal bleeding and portal hypertension: much to learn, much to explore. *Endoscopy* 2002; 34: 119–28.

Binmoeller KF, Soehendra N. 'Super glue'; the answer to variceal bleeding and fundal varices? *Endoscopy* 1995; 27: 392–6.

Boyce GA, Boyce HW. *Endoscopic Management of Gastrointestinal Tumors. Gastrointestinal Endoscopy Clinics of North America*, Vol. 2(3) (series ed. Sivak MV). Philadelphia: WB Saunders, 1992.

Carr-Locke DA, Al-Kawas F, Branch MH *et al.* Bipolar and multipolar accessories. *Gastrointest Endosc* 1996; 43: 779–82.

Carr-Locke DA, Branch MS, Byrne WJ *et al.* Botulinum toxin therapy in gastrointestinal endoscopy. *Gastrointest Endosc* 1998; 47: 569–72.

Carr-Locke DA, Conn MI, Faigel DO. Developments in laser technology. *Gastrointest Endosc* 1998; 48: 711–16.

Chung SCS, Leung JWC, Sung JY, Lo KK, Li AKC. Infection or heat probe for bleeding ulcer. *Gastroenterology* 1991; 100: 33–7.

Cook DJ, Guyatt GH, Salena BJ, Laine LA. Endoscopic therapy for acute nonvariceal upper gastrointestinal hemorrhage; a meta-analysis. *Gastroenterology* 1992; 102: 139–48.

D'Amico G, Pagliaro L, Bosch J. The treatment of portal hypertension: a meta-analytic review. *Hepatology* 1995; 22: 332.

Endoscopic band ligation of varices. *Gastrointest Endosc* 1998; 47: 573–5.

Esophageal dilation. *Gastrointest Endosc* 1998; 48: 702–4.

Filipi CJ, Lehman GA, Rothstein RI *et al.* Transoral, flexible endoscopic suturing for treatment of GERD: a multicenter trial. *Gastrointest Endosc* 2001; 63: 416–22.

Freeman ML, Cass OW, Peine CJ, Onstad GR. The non-bleeding visible vessel versus the sentinel clot: national history and risk of rebleeding. *Gastrointest Endosc* 1993; 39: 359–66.

Goff JS. Gastroesophageal varices: pathogenesis and therapy of acute bleeding. *Gastroenterol Clin North Am* 1993; 22: 779–800.

Guideline for the management of ingested foreign bodies. *Gastrointest Endosc* 1995; 42: 622–5.

Imperiale TE, Chalasani N. A meta-analysis of endoscopic variceal ligation for primary prophylaxis of esophageal variceal bleeding. *Hepatology* 2001; 33: 802–7.

Iwase H, Maeda O, Shimada M *et al.* Endoscopic ablation with cyanoacrylate glue for isolated gastric variceal bleeding. *Gastrointest Endosc* 2001; 53: 585–92.

Jalan R, Hayes PC. UK guidelines on the management of variceal haemorrhage in cirrhotic patients. *Gut* 2000; 46(Suppl 3-4): 1–15.

Kimmey MB, Al-Kawas F, Burnett DA *et al.* Electrocautery use in patients with implanted cardiac devices. *Gastrointest Endosc* 1994; 40(6): 794–5.

Kimmey MB, Al-Kawas F, Gannan RM. Balloon dilation of gastrointestinal tract strictures. *Gastrointest Endosc* 1995; 42: 608–11.

Laine L, Peterson WL. Bleeding peptic ulcer. *N Engl J Med* 1994; 331: 717–27.

Laine L, El-Newihi HM, Migikovsky B *et al.* Endoscopic ligation compared with sclerotherapy for treatment of bleeding esophageal varices. *Ann Intern Med* 1993; 119: 1–7.

Laine L, Stein C, Sharma V. Randomized comparison of ligation versus ligation plus sclerotherapy in patients with bleeding esophageal varices. *Gastroenterol* 1996; 110: 529–33.

Leiper K, Morris AI. Treatment of oesophago-gastric tumors. *Endoscopy* 2002; 34: 139–45.

Lightdale CJ. Staging of esophageal cancer: endoscopic ultrasonography. *Semin Oncol* 1994; 21: 438–46.

Lo GH, Lai KH, Cheng JS *et al.* Emergency banding ligation versus sclerotherapy for the control of active bleeding from esophageal varices. *Hepatology* 1997; 25: 1101–4.

McBride MA, Ergun GA. *The endoscopic management of esophageal strictures.* In: *Gastrointestinal Endoscopy Clinics of North America* (series ed. Sivak MV). WB Saunders 1994; 4(3): 595–621.

National Institutes of Health Consensus Conference. Therapeutic endoscopy and bleeding ulcers. *Gastrointest Endosc* 1990; 36: S1–S65.

Pasricha PJ, Fleischer DE, Kalloo AN. Endoscopic perforations of the upper digestive tract; a review of their pathogenesis, prevention and management. *Gastroenterology* 1994; 106: 787–802.

Pass HI. Photodynamic therapy in oncology: mechanisms and clinical use. *J Natl Cancer Inst* 1993; 85: 443–56.

Payne-James JJ, Spiller RC, Misiewicz JJ, Silk DBA. Use of ethanol-induced tumor necrosis to palliate dysphagia in patients with esophagogastric cancer. *Gastrointest Endosc* 1990; 36: 43–6.

Ponsky JL. *Percutaneous Endoscopic Gastrostomy. Gastrointestinal Endoscopy Clinics of North America*, Vol. 2(2) (series ed. Sivak MV). Philadelphia: WB Saunders, 1992.

Quinn PG, Connors PJ. *The role of upper gastrointestinal endoscopy in foreign body removal.* In: *Gastrointestinal Endoscopy Clinics of North America* (series ed. Sivak MV). Philadelphia: WB Saunders, 1994; 4(3): 571–93.

Rollhauser C, Fleischer DE. Nonvariceal upper gastrointestinal bleeding. *Endoscopy* 2002; 34: 111–18.

Sarin SK, Gupta R. Endoscopic ligation plus sclerotherapy: two plus two make only three! *Gastrointest Endosc* 1999; 50: 129–33.

Sarin SK, Govil A, Jain AK *et al.* Prospective randomized trial of endoscopic sclerotherapy versus variceal band ligation for esophageal varices: influence on gastropathy, gastric varices and variceal recurrence. *J Hepatol* 1997; 26: 826–32.

Vermeijden JR, Bartelsman JFWM, Fockens P *et al.* Self-expanding metal stents for palliation of esophagocardial malignancies. *Gastrointest Endosc* 1995; 41: 58–63.

Webb W. Management of foreign bodies of the upper gastrointestinal tract. *Gastroenterology* 1988; 94: 204–16.

Colonoscopy and Flexible Sigmoidoscopy

6

HISTORY

The history of colonoscopy started in 1958 in Japan with Matsunaga's intracolonic use of the gastrocamera under fluoroscopic control, and subsequently Niwa's development of the 'sigmocamera'. Not surprisingly, these instruments had application only in the hands of pioneer enthusiasts. Following Hirschowitz's development of the fiber-optic bundle in 1957–60 for use in prototype side-viewing gastroscopes, several colorectal enthusiasts started developments. The first was Overholt in the USA, who started on prototypes in 1961, performed the first fiber-optic flexible sigmoidoscopy in 1963, and finally introduced a commercial forward-viewing short 'fiberoptic coloscope' in 1966 (American Cystoscope Manufacturers Inc.). Meanwhile, Fox in the UK and Provenzale and Revignas in Italy had achieved imaging of the proximal colon with passive fiber-optic viewing bundles or side-viewing gastroscopes inserted up a radiologically inserted tube or pulled up by a swallowed transintestinal 'guide string and pulley' system. The West was surprised by the production in 1969 by Japanese engineers (Olympus Optical and Machida) of remarkably effective colonoscopes, which combined the precise two-way angulation and torque-stable shaft of the latest gastrocameras with superior fiber-optic bundles. Initially limitations of Japanese glass-fiber technology restricted angulation to around 90° (due to fragile fibers) and the angle of view to 70°. Niwa, in Japan, described gastric snare polypectomy in 1970, and snaring of colon polyps was pioneered in 1971 by Deyhle in Europe and Shinya in the USA.

Four-way acutely angulating instruments were introduced in the mid-1970s, then the video-endoscope in 1983 (Welch-Allyn, USA). Although small-scale colonoscope production continued for a time in the USA, Germany, Russia and China, the combined mechanical, optical and electronic know-how of the Japanese camera manufacturers now controls the market.

INDICATIONS AND LIMITATIONS

Indications and other methods

The place of colonoscopy in clinical practice depends on local circumstances and available endoscopic expertise. Although colonoscopy is considered the 'gold standard' exam, 'virtual' computed tomography (CT) colography or double-contrast barium enema (DCBE) alone may be considered by some to be adequate in 'low-yield' patients with constipation or functional symptoms, where the result is expected to be normal or likely to show only diverticular disease. Flexible sigmoidoscopy similarly, on grounds of logistics, safety and patient acceptability, has a significant role in clinically selected patients with minor symptoms and is being considered for population screening in countries without the resources to offer total colonoscopy.

Double-contrast barium enema (DCBE), in spite of its limitations, remains a safe way (one perforation per 25 000 examinations) of showing the configuration of the colon, the presence of diverticular disease and the absence of strictures or large lesions. Where colonoscopy services are overstretched, barium enema may be used in 'low yield' patients—those with pain, altered bowel habit or constipation; it also shows extramural leaks or fistulae, which are invisible to the endoscopist. With some justification, the outmoded technique of single-contrast enema was described by Gilbertsen as 'an excellent way of showing inoperable cancer'. Even high-quality DCBE has limitations, including the ability to miss large lesions because of overlapping loops (particularly in the sigmoid region), to misinterpret between solid stool and neoplasm or between spasm and strictures, with particular inaccuracy for flat lesions such as angiodysplasia or minor inflammatory change and small (2–5 mm) polyps.

CT colography ('virtual colonoscopy') is poised to overtake barium enema, with the advantages of being quicker and not filling the colon with dense contrast medium. CT colography similarly requires obsessional review of black and white images, and the visual opinion of the radiologist or technologist performing it. A few patients who are very difficult to colonoscope for reasons of anatomy or postoperative adhesions may be best examined by combining limited left-sided colonoscopy—the most challenging area for imaging but with the highest yield of significant pathology—with virtual colography or barium enema to demonstrate the proximal colon. Virtual colography has the advantage that it can be performed before or after colonoscopy and with the same bowel preparation.

Colonoscopy or flexible sigmoidoscopy achieves more than contrast radiology or virtual colography because of greater accuracy and its biopsy and therapeutic capabilities. Color view and biopsy makes total colonoscopy particularly relevant to patients with bleeding, anemia, bowel frequency or diarrhea. Flexible sigmoidoscopy alone may be sufficient for some patients, such as those with left iliac fossa pain. Because of near pinpoint accuracy and therapy, colonoscopy scores for any patient at increased risk for cancer—in whom detection and removal of all adenomas is important for the patient's future. Colonoscopy is thus the method of choice for many clinical indications and for cancer

High-yield indications	Low-yield indications
Anemia/bleeding/occult blood loss	Constipation
Persistent diarrhea	Flatulence
Inflammatory disease assessment	Altered bowel habit
Genetic cancer risk	Pain
Abnormality on imaging	
Therapy	

Table 6.1 Colonoscopy: indications and yield.

surveillance examinations and follow-up (Table 6.1). Endoscopy is also particularly useful in the postoperative patient, either to inspect in close-up (and biopsy if necessary) any deformity at the anastomosis or to avoid the difficulties of achieving adequate distension that leakage from a stoma presents for the imager.

Combined procedures (colonoscopy and virtual colography or DCBE) have potential advantages. If carbon dioxide (CO_2) insufflation is used for colonoscopy or flexible sigmoidoscopy, the colon will be absolutely deflated within 10–15 minutes and DCBE can follow immediately. Whereas air distension insufflation is a routine part of virtual colography, making it an ideal procedure to combine with colonoscopy, DCBE can be made difficult if the proximal colon is already air-filled and so difficult to coat adequately with barium. Colonoscopic biopsies with standard-sized forceps are no contraindication to distending the colon for DCBE or CT colography; prior pedunculated polypectomy should not be either. Larger biopsies or sessile polypectomy contraindicate using distension pressure, DCBE adding the potential danger of causing barium peritonitis—which can be fatal.

Limitations

There are limitations of colonoscopy. Incomplete examination can be due to inadequate bowel preparation, looping, inadequate hand-skills or an obstructing lesion, for example. A recent UK audit showed a completion rate of 75% (much lower in some centers). The lack of definite landmarks, unless the ileo-cecal valve is reached and identified, means that gross errors in colonoscopic localization are possible even for expert endoscopists. Any colonoscopist needs to be aware of the potential for blind spots, where it is possible to miss very large lesions, especially in the cecum, around acute bends and in the rectal ampulla. Colonoscopic examination, rigorously performed, can probably approach 90% accuracy for small lesions, but will never be 100%. A 'back to back' colonoscopy series, in which the patient was twice colonoscoped by two expert endoscopists, showed only 15% miss rate for polyps under 1 cm diameter. Every colonoscopist has experienced the chagrin of seeing a large polyp during insertion, but missing it entirely during withdrawal when the colon is crumpled after straightening it with the scope.

Hazards, complications and unplanned events

Colonoscopy is certainly more hazardous than barium studies (one perforation per 1700 colonoscopic examinations in published series against one perforation per 25 000 barium enemas). CT colography is certain to be safer still. Many published colonoscopy complication series, however, include early experience with outdated instruments and are certainly too pessimistic. There has been only a single perforation during diagnostic examinations by all those performing colonoscopies at St Mark's Hospital during the past 20 000 diagnostic colonoscopies. However, this is the experience of a specialist hospital and, whilst showing the potential for the technique, is not representative of what may be happening generally. Unskilled endoscopists needing to use heavy sedation or general anesthesia to cover up ineptitude are likely to run greater risks; it should not be considered a disgrace occasionally to abandon a tough colonoscopy in favor of CT colography.

Instrument shaft or tip perforations are usually due to inexperience and the use of excessive force when pushing in or pulling out. In a pathologically fixed, severely ulcerated or necrotic colon, however, forces that would be safe in a normal colon may be hazardous. Either the tip of the instrument or a loop formed by its shaft can perforate. Shaft loop perforations are characteristically larger than expected, so, if in doubt, surgery should be advised. When surgery has been performed soon after apparently uneventful colonoscopy, small tears have been seen in the ante-mesenteric serosal aspect of the colon, or hematomas found in the mesentery. In other cases the spleen has been avulsed during straightening maneuvers when the tip is hooked around the splenic flexure.

Air pressure perforations include 'blow-outs' of diverticula, 'pneumoperitoneum' and ileo-cecal perforation following colonoscopy limited to the sigmoid colon. Surprisingly high air pressures result if the scope tip is impacted in a diverticulum or if insufflation is excessive, for instance when trying to distend and pass a stricture or segment of severe diverticular disease. Use of CO_2 insufflation removes these serious sequelae, since it is so rapidly absorbed. Diverticula are thin walled and have also been perforated with biopsy forceps or by the instrument tip; it is surprisingly easy to confuse a large diverticular orifice with the bowel lumen.

Hypotensive episodes and even cardiac or respiratory arrest can be provoked by the combination of oversedation and the intense vagal stimulus of forceful or prolonged colonoscopy. Hypoxia is particularly likely in elderly patients, but should be a thing of the past now that pulse oximetry (or CO_2 capnography) is routinely used and nasal oxygen given prophylactically to elderly, ill or sedated patients.

Prophylactic antibiotics are only important in well-defined groups of patients, as has been mentioned elsewhere (see pp. 28–29): those with heart valve replacements, immunosuppressed or immunodepressed patients, and those with recent vascular grafts or previous infective endocarditis. Gram-negative septicemia can result from instrumentation (especially in neonates or the elderly) and unexplained postprocedure pyrexia or collapse should be investigated with blood cultures and managed appropriately.

Therapeutic procedures will inevitably cause occasional complications, including dilations (6% perforations in our series), electrocoagulation of bleeding points or sessile polypectomies. These are remarkably infrequent compared with the morbidity and mortality considered acceptable for surgery. To generalize (and perhaps exaggerate), endoscopic misadventure risks surgery; surgical misadventure risks death. The endoscopist should therefore be on guard that problems *can* occur and should only undertake therapeutic procedures with the knowledge and cooperation of a backup surgical team. Fatalities have also been reported after colonoscopic perforation followed by unnecessary surgery (rather than relying on conservative management with antibiotic cover). The decision whether or not to operate after a complication can be a subtle one, but the maxim should be 'if in doubt operate'; the surgeon consulted needs to be aware of the particular endoscopic circumstances. Most therapeutic perforations will be localized and occur in a well-prepared colon, so they may sometimes be considered for conservative management in the first resort. For instance, perforation following 'point electrocoagulation' of an angiodysplasia in the cecum has a reasonable chance of sealing off spontaneously (with the patient immobilized and on antibiotics). By contrast, an unexplained perforation after a difficult and forceful colonoscopy, especially if bowel preparation was poor, indicates exploratory surgery because there may be an extensive rent in the colon.

Safety during colonoscopy comes from gentle technique and avoiding pain (or oversedation, which masks the pain response, as well as contributing pharmacological hazards). Before starting a colonoscopy it is impossible to know if there are adhesions, whether the bowel is easily distensible and whether its mesenteries are free-floating or fixed; pain is the only warning that the bowel or its attachments are being unreasonably strained. The endoscopist must respect any protest from the patient. A mild groan in a sedated patient may be equivalent to a scream of pain without sedation. Moreover, it is hazardous to give repeated doses of sedatives intravenously, effectively anesthetizing the patient without an anesthetist being present; it is safer in such cases to abandon and reschedule as a formal anesthetic procedure. Total colonoscopy is *not* always technically possible, even for experts. If there is a history of abdominal surgery or sepsis, or if the instrument feels fixed and the patient is in pain, the correct course is usually to stop. The experienced endoscopist learns to take time, to be obsessional in steering correctly, to be prepared to withdraw from any difficult situation and if necessary to try again. Too often the beginner has a relentless 'crash and dash' approach, and may be insensitive to the patient's pain because it occurs so often.

Despite its potential hazards, skilled colonoscopy is amazingly *safe*; it is certainly justified by its clinical yield and the high morbidity of colonic surgery (which would often be the alternative). For the less skilled endoscopist, partnership with CT colography in 'difficult' cases should reduce the risks—with re-referral to an expert if pathology is found.

Informed consent

Obtaining full informed patient consent is essential before an invasive procedure such as colonoscopy, with the potential for complications. The patient should understand the rationale for undergoing the procedure, its benefits, risks, limitations and alternatives, and have an opportunity to ask the doctor any questions. Precise approaches to the explanation of risks vary from country to country, and should probably be tailored to some extent to the perceived insights and anxieties of the individual patient. Some patients wish to know everything, some would be distressed to have scary and unlikely minutiae (such as 'the unlikely possibility of death') spelled out to them. Any possible complication with an incidence greater than $1:100$ or $1:200$ should certainly be explained, so that a frank discussion of the 'pluses and minuses' of anticipated therapeutic procedures such as removal of large sessile polyps or dilation of strictures should be mandatory. Ideally the endoscopist quotes personal figures and experience.

It is logical to mention to all adult patients the remote possibility of *delayed bleeding* occurring for up to 10 days postprocedure, in case a polyp is found incidentally during colonoscopy and is judged to require removal (even though the procedure is scheduled as 'diagnostic'). Most patients will acquiesce immediately, but a commonsense discussion of practicalities is relevant. A patient about to have a holiday in remote parts or organizing a family wedding may be disinclined to take any risk whatever—and would justifiably be aggrieved should a complication occur.

Contraindications and infective hazards

There are few patients in whom colonoscopy is contraindicated. Any patient who might otherwise be considered for diagnostic laparotomy because of colonic disease is fit for colonoscopy, and colonoscopy is often undertaken in very poor risk cases in the hope of avoiding surgery.

For 3 months *after myocardial infarction,* it is unwise to perform colonoscopy due to the risk of dysrhythmias. There is no contraindication to colonoscopy (without fluoroscopy) during pregnancy, although, on commonsense grounds, it might be best avoided in those with a history of miscarriage. In any acute and severe inflammatory process (ulcerative, Crohn's or ischemic colitis) when abdominal tenderness suggests an increased risk of perforation, colonoscopy should only be undertaken with good reason and extreme care. If large and deep ulcers are seen, the bowel wall may be weakened and it may be wise to limit or abandon the examination. In the chronic stage after irradiation colitis, especially a year or more after exposure, the bowel can be perforated even without excessive force; if insertion proves difficult it may be wiser to withdraw.

Colonoscopy is absolutely contraindicated during and for 2–3 weeks after an episode of acute diverticulitis, due to the risk of perforation from the localized abscess or cavity. It should not be performed, or only with the greatest care and minimal insufflation, in any patient with marked abdominal tenderness, peritonism or peritonitis. Possible septicemia or infectivity are a consideration in certain patients. Passage of the colonoscope (and indeed any other investigation involving instrumentation or air or barium insufflation), causes transient release of bowel organisms into the bloodstream and peritoneal cavity. This constitutes a relative contraindication to endoscopy of patients with known ascites or on peritoneal dialysis. They, and patients with heart-valve replacements, and also marasmic infants or immunosuppressed or immunodepressed adults, should be protected by the prior administration of antibiotics (see p. 29). There is no contraindication to the examination of infected patients (e.g. patients with infectious diarrhea or hepatitis) because all normal organisms and viruses should be inactivated by routine cleaning and disinfection procedures. Mycobacterial spores, however, require a much longer period so, after the examination of suspected tuberculosis patients and before and after the examination of AIDS patients (who are susceptible to, and possible carriers of, mycobacteria) a 60 minutes soak of the instrument in glutaraldehyde is recommended (see Chapter 2).

Careful history-taking by nurse or doctor is essential during the process of obtaining information and consent, including relevant previous medical history and current medications. For obvious reasons, medications such as anticoagulants or insulin may affect management. A cardiac pacemaker contraindicates use of the 3-D imager or argon plasma coagulation (APC).

PATIENT PREPARATION

Most patients can manage bowel preparation at home, present for colonoscopy and walk out shortly afterwards. Management routines depend on national, organizational and individual factors. Overall management is influenced, among other things, by:

• cost;
• facilities available;
• type of bowel preparation and sedation used;
• age and state of the individual patient;
• potential for major therapeutic procedures;
• availability of adequate facilities and nursing staff for day-care and recovery.

Experienced colonoscopists in private practice or large units are motivated to organize streamlined day-case routines, even for patients with large polyps. Some nationalities (Dutch, Japanese) do not expect sedation whereas others (British, American) frequently insist on it. In countries with sufficient anesthesiologists (France, Italy, Australia) a full general anesthetic can, regrettably, become the norm. These variables result in an extraordinary spectrum of performance around the world, from the many skilled colonoscopists who require patients for less than an hour on a 'walk-in, walk-out' basis in an office or day-care unit, to others with less experience and a traditional hospital background who feel that many hours in hospital, or even an overnight stay, are essential.

Colonoscopy can be made quick and easy for the majority of patients. This requires both a reasonably planned day-care facility and an endoscopist with the confidence and skill to work gently and reasonably fast. Some flexibility of approach is wise. A very few patients are better admitted before or after the procedure; the very old, sick and very constipated may need professional supervision during bowel preparation. Frail patients may merit overnight observation afterwards if their domestic circumstances are not supportive or they live far away. We admit a few patients for polypectomy, especially if the lesion is very large and sessile or if the patient has a bleeding diathesis or is on anticoagulants or antiplatelet medications (aspirin, dipyrinamide, etc.). However, even such patients, providing they live near good medical support services and have been fully informed about what to do in a crisis, can often be justifiably managed on an outpatient basis, since complications are rare—and can be 'delayed', occurring several days after the procedure.

Bowel preparation

A doctor, nurse or other informed team member should talk to the patient at the time of booking to explain the procedure, and the importance of successful bowel preparation. Most people who haven't had colonoscopy subsequently admit that the anticipation of it, including fear of indignity, of a painful experience or the possible findings, is worse than the reality of the procedure itself. Anything that will justifiably cheer them up beforehand, whilst ensuring understanding and also compliance with dietary modification and bowel preparation, is extremely worthwhile. Minutes spent in explanation and motivation may prevent a prolonged, unpleasant and inaccurate examination due to bad preparation. The patient needs to know that a properly prepared colon looks as clean and easy to examine as the mouth—whereas poor preparation leads to a degradingly unpleasant and inaccurate examination.

Limited preparation

Enemas alone are usually effective for limited colonoscopy or flexible sigmoidoscopy in the 'normal' colon. The patient need not diet and typically has one or two disposable phosphate enemas (e.g. Fleet Phospho-soda®, Fletchers', Microlax), self-administered or given by nursing staff. Examination can be performed shortly after evacuation occurs—usually within 10–15 minutes—so that there is no time for more proximal bowel contents to descend. The colon can often be perfectly prepared to the transverse colon in younger subjects (in babies phosphate enemas are contraindicated because of the risk of phosphatemia). Note that patients with any tendency to faint or with functional bowel symptoms (pain, flatulence, etc.) are more likely to have severe vasovagal problems after phosphate enemas; make sure they are supervised or have a call button, and that lavatory doors open from and towards the outside in case the patient should faint against the door.

Diverticular disease or stricturing require full bowel preparation even for a limited examination, because bowel preparation will be less effective and phosphate enemas less likely to work.

If obstruction is a possibility, peroral preparation is dangerous, even potentially fatal. In ileus or pseudo-obstruction, normal preparation simply does not work. One or more large-volume enemas are administered in such circumstances (up to 1 liter or more can be held by most colons). A contact laxative such as oxyphenisatin (300 mg) or a dose of bisacodyl can be added to the enema to improve evacuation (see below).

Full preparation

The object of full preparation is to cleanse the whole colon, especially the proximal parts, which are characteristically coated with surface residue after limited regimens. However, patients and colons vary. No single preparation regime predictably suits every patient, and it is often necessary to be prepared to adapt to individual needs. Constipated patients need extra preparation; those with severe colitis may be unfit to have anything other than a warm saline or tapwater enema. A preparation that has previously proved unpalatable, made the patient vomit or that failed is unlikely to be a success on another occasion—a different one should be substituted.

Diet

Dietary restriction is a crucial part of preparation. Iron preparations should be stopped at least 3–4 days before colonoscopy, since organic iron tannates produce an inky black and viscous stool, which interferes with inspection and is difficult to clear. Constipating agents should also be stopped 1–2 days before, but most other medications can be continued as usual, allowing for modification of anticoagulant regimens and the avoidance of aspirin, non-steroidal anti-inflammatory drugs (NSAIDs) and similar platelet-inhibiting agents, if possible, in those of polyp-bearing age.

The patient should have no indigestible or high-residue food for 24 hours before colonoscopy (avoiding muesli, fibrous vegetables, mushrooms, fruit, nuts, raisins, etc.). Staying for 24 hours on clear fluids is even better if the patient is compliant, but isn't really necessary. Soft foods that are easily digested (soups, omelettes, potato, cheese and ice-cream), are present in most menus and can be eaten up to (and including) lunch on the day preceding colonoscopy. Only supper and breakfast before colonoscopy need to be replaced with fluids. Tea or coffee (with some milk if wanted) can be drunk up to the last minute, any darkish fluid residue presenting no problem to the endoscopist. Fruit juices or beer are found by many to be easier to drink in large quantities than water, and white wine or (diluted!) spirits can also help morale during the fasting phase. However, *red wine is discouraged* because it contains iron and tannates and, when digested with other dietary tannates, causes the bowel contents to become black, sticky and offensive. Any other clear drink, water ices or sorbets (not blackcurrant), consommé (hot or cold), boiled sweets or peppermints can all be taken up to the last minute—there is no reason why anyone should feel ravenous or unduly deprived by the time of colonoscopy.

Written dietary instructions including these tips are well worthwhile, since many patients, anxious to get a good result, find it easier to follow specific instructions 'to the letter'. It also avoids unnecessary anxieties and telephone calls from the obsessional.

Oral lavage regimes

Oral lavage regimes of one kind or another are universally used, supplanting the traditional 'purge-plus-enema' approach because they are more effective and cause no pain. On the other hand, some patients will not, or cannot, drink the full 3–4 liter volumes of fluid required, experience uncomfortable distension, become nauseated or vomit, or simply dislike the taste of the chosen solution. Further work is needed to provide the ideal compromise—a powder that can be sent through the mail and dissolved to produce an acceptable volume of a pleasant-tasting combination of non-absorbed solutes and electrolytes, perhaps also containing a physiological gut activator and/or a prokinetic agent to speed transit.

Balanced electrolyte solutions are physiologically correct, including the requisite amount of sodium and potassium chloride and bicarbonate to avoid body losses. Unfortunately the taste of the additives (especially the KCl and Na_2SO_4) is inherently unpleasant. Normal (0.9%) saline alone is used by some centers; this has the advantage of being very cheap and easy to make up or send through the mail, but it is less 'physiological'.

PEG-electrolyte solution

Balanced electrolyte solution with polyethylene glycol solution (PEG)—more properly PEG-electrolyte solution—is very widely used. This is primarily because it has formal approval from the US Food and Drug Administration (FDA) (e.g. GoLytely®, Nulytely®, Colyte®, KleenPrep®, etc.) and comes with suitable flavorings, convenient packaging and is easily prescribed, but it is surprisingly expensive. Although the PEG component of a PEG-electrolyte mixture—often known as PEG preparation—contributes the majority of the packaged weight, volume and expense, it results in only a minority of the osmolality (sodium salts being, of physiological necessity, the important component). Even chilled, its taste is mildly unpleasant due to the Na_2SO_4, bicarbonate and KCl included to minimize body fluxes. Modification of the original formula (Nulytely®) by omitting Na_2SO_4 and reducing KCl, only slightly improves the taste. Patient acceptance of PEG-electrolyte oral preparation can be enhanced, without impairing results from the endoscopist's point of view, by the simple expedient of administering the 3–4 liters necessary in two half doses ('split administration'), with 2 liters drunk the evening before and 1–2 liters on the morning of the examination. There are conflicting reports about whether the addition of prokinetic agents or aperients improves results; the consensus is that it doesn't.

Mannitol

Mannitol (and similarly sorbitol or lactulose) is a disaccharide sugar for which the body has no absorptive enzymes. It is available as a very cheap white powder, looking and tasting similar to glucose, or as ready-made intravenous solutions (more expensive but easily available), which can be drunk. In solution mannitol presents an isosmotic fluid load at 5% (2–3 L) or a hypertonic purge at 10% (1 L) with a corresponding loss of electrolyte and body fluid during the resulting diarrhea, although this is only of concern in the elderly and normally can be rapidly reversed by drinking. The solution's sweetness can be nauseous to those without a sweet tooth, although this is much reduced by chilling and adding lemon juice or other flavorings. Children, in particular, tend to vomit it back. Mannitol solution alone (1 L of 10% mannitol drunk iced over 30 minutes, followed by 1 L of tapwater) is a useful way of achieving rapid bowel preparation (in 2–3 hours) for those requiring urgent colonoscopy or, as 2 L of 5% solution, avoids active aperients in patients with active colitis.

There is a potential *explosion hazard* after mannitol, because colonic bacteria possess the necessary enzymes to metabolize mannitol and similar carbohydrates to form explosive concentrations of hydrogen. If carbohydrates have been used in preparation, electrosurgery is hazardous unless CO_2 insufflation has been used, or all colonic gas is conscientiously exchanged several times by aspiration and reinsufflation of room air.

Magnesium salts

Magnesium citrate and other magnesium salts are very poorly absorbed, acting as an 'osmotic purge' and known, since Roman times, as Vichy and other similar 'spa' waters, for their gently cathartic properties. Picolax®, a proprietary combination, produces both magnesium citrate (from magnesium oxide and citric acid) and bisacodyl (from bacterial action on sodium picosulfate), tastes acceptable and works well in most patients. Providing enough fluid is drunk, no enema is needed. Magnesium citrate alone (1 L of 10% solution, or 100 g magnesium oxide and citric acid as powder) seems to be as effective and is more readily available. When made up from powder substantial frothing and release of heat occurs, so a large jug should be used and the solution cooled with ice cubes when fully dissolved and clear. Some people find the result pleasantly lemon-tasting, others find it very bitter—which can be countered by adding sugar, sweetener and/or any flavoring or cordial, then drinking a beaker-full at a time, followed by other preferred clear fluids. Painless diarrhea can be expected within 2–3 hours. For the seriously constipated, magnesium sulfate, although unpleasant-tasting, is highly effective if taken in repeated hourly doses (5 mL of crystals in 200 mL hot water, followed by juice and other fluids) and guaranteed eventually 'to move mountains'.

Sodium phosphate

Sodium phosphate, presented as a flavored half-strength orally administered equivalent of the phosphate enema (Fleet's Phospho-soda®), has received numerous good reports when trialed against PEG-electrolyte preparation. It proves to be as effective as PEG-electrolyte solution but significantly more acceptable to patients, principally because the volume ingested is only 90 mL. It must be followed by at least 1 liter of other clear fluids of choice—water, juices, lager, etc. No large trial has been made against other apparently very acceptable and effective regimes—such as the senna/magnesium citrate combination.

Routine for taking oral preparations

Low-residue diet instructions should have been followed. The patient is preferably supplied with petroleum jelly or barrier cream to avoid perianal soreness (colorless if possible to avoid endoscope lens contamination).

As mentioned above, large-volume PEG-electrolyte solutions are ideally split-administered in two doses, starting on the evening beforehand but with the remainder taken on the morning of the examination so that the cecal contents remain fluid. If an afternoon examination is scheduled, and the patient does not have a long distance to travel, both doses can be drunk on the day of examination. If in doubt, a purgative (such as senna, 4–6 tablets) can be also be taken at the previous bedtime in order to 'prime the pump'.

PEG-electrolyte solution should be drunk at a rate of around 1.5 L/h (250 mL/10 min initially). Chilling mannitol solution makes it taste much less sweet; cooling PEG-electrolyte solution also improves palatability but may overcool the drinker too. Adding sugar-containing flavoring agents, such as fruit cordials, to PEG-electrolyte solution is discouraged on the theoretical basis that increased sodium absorption could occur, but using 'diabetic' cordials would avoid this. Sodium phosphate solution is easily downed with a 'chaser' of some more pleasant drink, and then 1 liter or more of any fluid to follow in the next hour or two.

The patient should be encouraged to carry on with normal activities, rather than sitting still during the drinking period, in order to encourage transit. Drinking should stop temporarily if nausea or uncomfortable distension occurs. Bowel actions should start within about an hour, returns are often clear by 2–3 hours and colonoscopy can sometimes be started 1–2 hours later. The endoscopist may have to aspirate large quantities of fluid during the examination but the patient is spared the dietary changes, cramps and occasional vasovagal effects of a purge regimen. The result is usually excellent providing that the whole volume (or nearly all) has been drunk. In the 10% of patients where nausea or vomiting prevents this the proximal colon surface can be badly coated with residue.

Purgative/'mag. cit.' preparations

This compromise regime combines a purge and osmotic lavage, is easily taken, pleasant-tasting to most people and almost universally effective. The principle is to cause minimal interruption to the patient's normal routine, so allowing a normal working day before colonoscopy. Because there is less 'fluid overload' than with a PEG-electrolyte preparation, another essential is that the final dose of magnesium citrate must be taken only a few hours before exam. It takes only about 8 hours for colonic water absorption to reform ileal effluent into solid stool; it is therefore disastrous if preparation stops the previous evening—this will result in sticky and opaque residue coating the cecum.

The purgative dose is taken to 'prime the pump' and trigger evacuation following 24 hours of a soft, low-residue diet (as described above), up to and including lunch on the day preceding exam. Some people respond to laxatives in 1–2 hours and others take as much as 8–10 hours, so exact timing is problematic. If the patient is not to miss work, but be able to travel home without risk of accident and later get some overnight sleep, the best compromise is for the laxative to be taken at 3–5 pm on the pre-exam day. However, for an afternoon colonoscopy, the purge can be taken at bedtime in the expectation that there will be no action during sleep—until the gut reactivates in the morning.

Purges. Castor oil (30–40 mL) was the traditional agent used before surgery and contrast studies, but is disliked by most patients because of its aftertaste and oily texture. Senna preparations can be sweet and chocolate-flavored (granules or syrup) and work equally well, providing a large dose is given (140 mg of sennosides—equivalent to six or more senna tablets). Two bisacodyl tablets are easier to take, tasteless but highly effective, and are probably the purge of choice.

The patient must anticipate that the evening before colonoscopy will be a fluid experience—input and output. Other social events should not be scheduled, but there will be plenty of time for television or reading between 'calls'. With alcoholic or other beverages the evening can be passed not unpleasantly. The first dose of magnesium citrate can be mixed (see above) and taken around 5.30–6.30 pm, leaving time for a further half dose at 9–10 pm before bed. For morning colonoscopies the remaining half dose must be taken on rising at 6–7 am, with coffee, tea or other fluids to follow; whereas for late morning or afternoon exams the whole second magnesium citrate dose (even both doses) can be taken on the morning of examination. Since magnesium simply overloads the intestinal absorptive mechanism and produces a gentle 'tidal wave' without particular urgency—and rarely any cramps or urgency—this essential final dose often appears to the patient to have little effect, but guarantees a clean cecum for the endoscopist.

Bowel preparation in special circumstances

Children accept pleasant-tasting oral preparations such as senna syrup or magnesium citrate very well. Drinking large volumes is less well accepted, and mannitol may cause nausea or vomiting. The childhood colon normally evacuates easily except, paradoxically, in colitis patients who prove perversely difficult to prepare properly. Small babies may be almost completely prepared with oral fluids plus a saline enema. Phosphate enemas are contraindicated in babies because of the possibility of hyperphosphatemia.

Colitis patients require special care, during and after preparation. Relapses of inflammatory bowel disease are said occasionally to occur after over-vigorous bowel preparation, although they can also be provoked by simple distension during an unprepared barium enema, which perhaps suggests that the cause is mechanical rather than chemical. Magnesium citrate, senna preparations, mannitol, saline or balanced PEG-electrolyte solutions are all generally well tolerated, and the latter is favored in patients with diarrhea from active colitis. A simple tapwater or saline enema will clear the distal colon sufficiently for limited colonoscopy. Patients with severe colitis are unlikely to need colonoscopy at all, since plain abdominal X-ray (or if necessary an unprepared contrast study) will usually give enough information. For severely ill patients even a barium enema is risky and colonoscopy positively contraindicated, due to the potential for perforation. When the indication for colonoscopy in a colitis patient is to exclude cancer or to reach the terminal ileum to help in differential diagnosis, full and vigorous preparation is necessary. A patient fit enough for total colonoscopy is fit for full bowel preparation, which is essential because inflammatory change often makes the proximal colon difficult to prepare properly.

Constipated patients often need extra bowel preparation. This is very difficult to achieve in patients with true megacolon or Hirschsprung's disease, in whom colonoscopy should be avoided if at all possible. Constipated patients should continue any habitually taken purgatives in addition to the colonoscopy preparation, preferably in large doses for several days beforehand. The principle is to achieve regular soft bowel actions during the days before taking the main purge, if necessary using additional doses of magnesium citrate/sulfate, etc. Larger than standard doses of senna or other purgatives are unlikely to produce any extra effect, but frequent doses of magnesium salts and large volumes of fluid are guaranteed to be effective (see above), providing there is no obstruction.

Colostomy patients are as difficult to prepare as normal subjects (and often more so). The preparation regimen should not be reduced just because the colon is shorter; if anything it should be increased, with a prior 'pump-priming' maximal dose of senna on the night before. Oral preparation with one of the lavage regimens described above is well tolerated, whereas enemas/colostomy washouts are tedious and difficult for nursing staff to perform satisfactorily, unless the patient is accustomed to this and used to performing it personally.

Stomas, pouches and ileo-rectal anastomoses present few problems. Ileostomies are self-emptying and normally need no preparation other than perhaps a few hours of fasting and clear fluid intake. Ileo-anal pelvic pouches can be managed either by saline enema or by reduced oral lavage. After ileo-rectal anastomosis, the small intestine can adapt and enlarge to an amazing degree within some months of surgery, so that if the object of the examination is to examine the small intestine, full oral preparation should be given. For a limited look, a saline or tapwater enema is usually enough; stimulant enemas will sometimes elicit a vasovagal response.

Defunctioned bowel, for instance the distal loop of a 'double-barrelled' colostomy, always contains a considerable amount of viscid mucus and inspissated cell debris, which will block the colonoscope. Conventional tapwater or saline rectal enemas or tube lavage through the colostomy are needed before examining a defunctioned bowel. Hypertonic (phosphate) or stimulant enemas will be less effective.

Active colonic bleeding modifies preparation since blood is a good purgative. Some patients requiring emergency colonoscopy may need no specific preparation at all, providing that examination is started during the phase of active bright-red bleeding. Posturing the patient during insertion of the instrument will shift the blood and create an air interface through which the instrument can be passed; changing to the right lateral position clears the proximal sigmoid and descending colon, which is otherwise a blood-filled sump. Actively bleeding patients requiring preparation for more accurate total colonoscopy are best managed by nasogastric tube or oral electrolyte/mannitol lavage. This allows examination within an hour or two and ensures that blood is washed out distal to the bleeding point, rather than carried proximally with enemas. Blood can be refluxed to the terminal ileum from a left colon source, which makes localization difficult unless it is being constantly washed downwards by a peroral high-volume preparation. Massively bleeding patients can be examined per-operatively with on-table colon lavage combining a cecostomy tube with a large-bore rectal suction tube (and bucket).

MEDICATION

Sedation and analgesia

All aspects of the procedure, including the medication options, should be explained when the colonoscopy booking is arranged. The patient should (whether by doctor, nurse or secretary) receive preliminary verbal and written explanation about bowel preparation and what to expect of the procedure. At this point some patients may judge (in wise countries where judgment is permitted) that they want full medication, others that they will hope to work normally or to drive afterwards. On arrival for colonoscopy, a few minutes of further explanation will reassure and calm most patients and allow the endoscopist to judge whether the particular individual is likely to require sedation, and if so how much. Most people tolerate some discomfort without resentment if they understand the reason for it. Few people expect to be semi-anesthetized for a visit to the dentist, but on the other hand they understandably expect the intensity and duration of any pain to be within 'acceptable limits'. Pain thresholds and individual attitudes to pain are not always easy to predict before colonoscopy, because tolerance of the (peculiarly unpleasant) dull quality of visceral pain varies so much. It is sensible to warn the patient that there may be some 'stomach ache' or feeling of 'gas distension' during the procedure, and to ask them to give feedback at once, rather than suffering in silence.

During a correctly performed colonoscopy, pain is experienced by the patient for only 20–30 seconds. Using moderate or no sedation, and employing the skills, changes of position and other 'tricks of the trade' described below, pain only occurs while looping up the sigmoid colon and passing the sigmoid–descending colon junction, before straightening out the instrument and stopping this 'stretch pain'. During the rest of a normal procedure there should, with luck and some hand-skills, be little more than a feeling of distension or the desire to pass flatus. It is worth pointing out to the patient that any pain is useful because it shows that a loop is forming, but is not dangerous and can usually be terminated in a few seconds (by straightening out the loop that is causing it).

The use of sedation has advantages and disadvantages. The unsedated or very lightly sedated patient can co-operate by changing position, needs no recovery period and can travel home unaided immediately. The colonoscopist is also forced to develop good, gentle insertion technique. On the other hand, some endoscopists who never employ sedation admit to only

70–80% success in performing total colonoscopy, presumably because some examinations were intolerable. If some degree of 'conscious sedation' is used (typically equivalent in effect to 2–3 glasses of wine or beer), the patient is more likely to find the examination tolerable, even enjoyable, or to have amnesia for it. The endoscopist can perhaps be more thorough in the knowledge that the patient is comfortable, and is also more likely to achieve total colonoscopy in a shorter time. However, with heavy sedation endoscopists can get away with ham-handed forcibly looping technique—a bad investment in the long term, less likely to achieve complete examinations, more likely to result in complications and more expensive in instrument repair bills. It is often said that it is dangerous to sedate, because the safety factor of pain is removed; this is not strictly true, providing that the endoscopist raises his own threshold of awareness as the patient's pain threshold is raised, responding to restlessness or changes of facial expression as a warning that tissues and attachments are being overstretched.

Most endoscopists use a balanced approach to sedation that will be affected by many factors, including personal experience and the individual patient's attitude. A relaxed patient with a short colon having a limited examination rarely needs sedation, but an anxious patient with a tortuous colon, severe diverticular disease, or a bad previous experience needs some protection. A very few patients have such a morbid fear of colonoscopy, such a low pain threshold or a known 'difficult' colon that it is justified to resort to light general anesthesia. General anesthesia is only likely to be hazardous when employed by an inexperienced colonoscopist, able to use brutal technique because the anesthetized patient cannot protest. However, even experienced endoscopists are more likely to 'push the limits' and tend to become more mechanistic when the patient is anesthetized and 'out of it'.

Nitrous oxide inhalation

Nitrous oxide/oxygen inhalation can be a useful 'half-way house' between no sedation and conventional intravenous sedation. The 50 : 50 nitrous oxide/oxygen mixture is self-administered by the patient, inhaling from a small cylinder fitted with a demand valve. Breathing the gas through a small single-use mouthpiece (Fig. 6.1) avoids the difficulties that can be experienced in getting a good fit with a face mask, and also the phobia that some patients feel for masks. Because of the possible teratogenicity of passively inhaled nitrous oxide to females of child-bearing age, a gas-scavenging system must be in place before routine use, but may be unnecessary for occasional usage.

The patient is shown how to inhale, then 'prebreathes' for a minute or so as the endoscopist prepares to start the procedure,

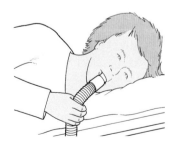

Fig. 6.1 Nitrous oxide/oxygen mixture is breathed through a mouthpiece.

with the intention of achieving gas saturation of the body fatty tissues. Thereafter it takes only 20–30 seconds of gas breathing, when needed, to obtain a 'high' that makes short-lived pain significantly more tolerable. Nitrous oxide/oxygen inhalation should prove useful for some flexible sigmoidoscopies and is sufficient for motivated patients having total colonoscopy by a skilled endoscopist. Scared patients, prolonged or difficult examinations, and examinations by inexpert endoscopists require conventional sedation.

Intravenous sedation

The ideal sedative regime for colonoscopy would last only 5–10 minutes, with a strong analgesic action but no respiratory depression or after-effects, allowing the patient to be comfortable yet accessible and able to change position during the procedure but then to recover rapidly afterwards. The nearest approach to the ideal is currently given by intravenous infusion, through an indwelling plastic cannula, of a benzodiazepine hypnotic such as midazolam (Versed® 1.25–5 mg maximum) or diazepam (Valium® or Diazemuls® 2.5–10 mg maximum) either alone or combined with a low dose of an opiate such as pethidine (meperidine 25–100 mg maximum). The benzodiazepine contributes anxiolytic, sedational and amnesic effects while the opiate contributes analgesia and, in the case of pethidine, a useful sense of euphoria. In general, only a small dose of benzodiazepine should be given unless the patient is very anxious. The initial injection is given slowly over a period of at least 1 minute, 'titrating' the dose to some extent by observing the patient's conscious state and ability to talk coherently—some patients merely become loquacious. A small initial starter dose makes it possible to judge during initial insertion through the sigmoid whether the rest of the procedure is likely to be easy or difficult, and whether the patient is pain-sensitive or not. Half dosage in total is used for older, sicker patients but the amount required is unpredictable; younger patients may tolerate maximal doses and remain (fairly) coherent. If in doubt it is safer to under-do the titration and give more later if necessary.

Use extra opiate rather than more benzodiazepine if extra medication is needed. Benzodiazepines make some patients even more restless and have no painkilling properties. Benzodiazepines and opiates potentiate each other, not only in effectiveness but also in side-effects such as depression of respiration and blood pressure, which can be sudden or gradual, and potentially serious. Pulse oximetry should therefore be routinely used. In many units nasal oxygen is routinely administered in all sedated patients—with the caveat that this is contraindicated in chronic obstructive airways disease (COAD), where CO_2 capnography would ideally be used.

Benzodiazepines have a useful mild smooth-muscle anti-spasmodic action as well as their anxiolytic effect. Diazepam (Valium®) is poorly soluble in water and the injectable form is therefore carried in a glycol solution that can be painful and cause thrombophlebitis, especially if administered into small veins. If a hand vein is to be used, and also for pediatric practice, it is better either to use water-soluble midazolam (Versed®) or diazepam in lipid emulsion (Diazemuls®, where available), both of which are less irritant. Midazolam causes a greater degree of amnesia, which can be useful to cover a traumatic experience but also 'wipes' any explanation of the findings, which must be repeated later on. It should be borne in mind that intravenous midazolam dosage should be half that of diazepam.

Opiates (pethidine notably) induce a useful sense of euphoria in addition to analgesic efficacy. Pethidine may cause local pain when administered through small veins, particularly in children, but this can largely be avoided by diluting the injection 1: 10 in water. Some endoscopists prefer to give pethidine (meperidine) intramuscularly 1 h beforehand. Pentazocine (Fortral®) is a weaker analgesic, more hallucinogenic and seems to have little to recommend it. Fentanyl (Sublimaze®) is a very short-lived opiate, but has the disadvantage of significant respiratory depressant effects without giving any sense of well-being.

Propofol (Diprivan®), a short-lived intravenous emulsion anesthetic agent, is widely used for colonoscopy in some countries (France, Germany, Australia) and sporadically in others. It should ideally be administered by an anesthetist because of the significant risk of marked respiratory depression but, with appropriate training and safeguards, has been employed by endoscopists alone. Its short duration of action—giving full recovery within about 30 minutes—is an advantage over excessive doses of conventional sedatives. On the other hand, the patient is rendered insensible and so unable to co-operate with changes of position or to give early warning of excessive pain. The routine use of propofol for all cases cannot therefore be recommended.

Antagonists

The availability of antagonists to benzodiazepines (flumazenil) and opiates (naloxone) is invaluable, providing a safety measure for occasions when inadvertent oversedation has occurred. Some endoscopists routinely administer antagonists (intravenously and/or intramuscularly) to reduce the recovery period, which suggests mainly that their 'routine' dosage regime is excessive. We use flumazenil extremely infrequently, but periodically administer naloxone intramuscularly on reaching the cecum in a patient who has requested or needed extra sedation. The patient is then conveniently awake by the time the examination is finished, without the risk of later 'rebound' re-sedation, which is reported after intravenous naloxone wears off.

Antispasmodics

Antispasmodics induce colonic relaxation for at least 5–10 minutes and help to optimize the view during examination of a hypercontractile colon. Either hyoscine N-butylbromide (Buscopan®) 20 mg IV (in countries where it can be prescribed) or glucagon 0.5–1 mg IV are effective The ocular side-effects of hyoscine may continue for several hours, and the patient should not drive if vision is impaired, although cholinesterase-inhibitor eye drops will rapidly restore normality. Fears about anticholinergics initiating glaucoma are misplaced because patients previously diagnosed are completely protected by their eye drops, and those with undiagnosed chronic glaucoma are best served by precipitating an acute attack, which will cause the diagnosis to be made. Glucagon is more expensive, but has no ocular or prostatic side-effects.

Intravenous antispasmodics have a relatively short duration of action, leading some endoscopists to give them when the colonoscope is fully inserted; experienced endoscopists, sure of a rapid procedure, may give them at the start. There is an unproven suspicion that the bowel is rendered more redundant and atonic by antispasmodics and will be more difficult to examine. To the contrary, we find that the view is improved and colonoscope insertion speeded up after using antispasmodics. Benzodiazepines have a weak antispasmodic effect, relaxing most colons except for those that are 'irritable' or spastic; in the unsedated patient therefore antispasmodics may be particularly helpful—and can also be a useful placebo for those who cannot have routine sedation because they need to drive home, but expect an 'injection' to cover the procedure.

Inflation with CO_2 avoids postprocedure problems in patients with functional bowel disorder or diverticular disease who may suffer from increased air retention, with the sudden onset of colic or abdominal discomfort an hour or more after the procedure when the pharmacological effects of the antispasmodics and sedation wear off.

Antibiotics

Bacteremia occurs while the instrument is being inserted through the sigmoid colon, as proven by studies in which multiple blood cultures are taken during colonoscopy. Both aerobic and anaerobic organisms can be released into the bloodstream at this time. Patients with ascites or on peritoneal dialysis have been reported to develop peritonitis following colonic instrumentation, presumably by transmural passage of bacteria as a result of local trauma. At-risk patients (see also pp. 28–29) (including those with heart-valve replacements, cyanotic heart disease, previous endocarditis or a recent aortic prosthesis) and immunosuppressed, severely neutropenic or gravely ill patients (especially immunocompromised infants) should have a suitable antibiotic combination administered beforehand so as to give therapeutic blood levels at the time of the procedure. A possible adult regimen is: ampicillin 3 g orally 1 hour beforehand—or 1 g in 2.5 mL 1% lidocaine (lignocaine) intramuscularly (IM) just beforehand—*plus* another 0.5 g orally 6 hours later and gentamicin 120 mg IM 1 hour before (or IV just beforehand). Alternatively give a single IV dose of gentamicin (80 mg) and ampicillin (500 mg) before premedication. Vancomycin (20 mg/kg by slow IV infusion over the 60 minutes prior to the procedure) can be substituted for ampicillin in patients with a history of penicillin sensitivity. Children under 10 years of age receive half the adult dose of amoxicillin and gentamicin—2 mg/kg body weight. In high-risk subjects it may be wise to continue antibiotics for up to 24–48 hours.

EQUIPMENT

Colonoscopy room

Most units perform colonoscopies in undesignated endoscopy rooms, because the only special requisite for colonoscopy is good ventilation, to overcome the evidence of occasional poor bowel preparation. In a few patients with particularly difficult and looping colons it has in the past been helpful to have access to X-ray facilities, particularly in teaching institutions. Three-dimensional (3D) imaging systems (see below), will perform the same function without X-rays.

Colonoscopes

Colonoscopes are engineered similarly to upper gastrointestinal endoscopes, but are longer, wider-diameter (for better twist or torque control) and have a more flexible shaft. The bending section of the colonoscope tip is also longer and so more gently curved, to avoid impaction in acute bends, such as the splenic flexure. Ideally, colonoscope control-body ergonomics and angulation controls will in future be modified (with a tracker ball or similar mechanism controlling power-steering facilities) so as to make one-handed steering and activation of the different controls and switches easier. Present control mechanisms are almost unchanged from those of early gastrocameras and gastroscopes and are far from ideal for the more finicky steering movements required during colonoscopy. Video-colonoscopes have largely eclipsed the use of fiber-optic instruments because they do not need to be held near the endoscopist's face, so have positional and hygienic advantages, and allow everyone to see, bringing all the benefits of high-resolution electronic image management. Nonetheless, a fiber-colonoscope can be used with a CCD 'video adaptor', with many of the same benefits.

The introduction of 'variable stiffness' instruments avoids the need to choose the 'right colonoscope for the job' at the stage of purchase or before starting examination of a particular patient—especially one known to have a long 'difficult' colon or severe adhesions. Long colonoscopes (165–180 cm) are able to reach the cecum even in redundant colons and so are our preferred routine choice of instrument (see also 'variable-stiffness colonoscopes' below). Intermediate-length instruments (130–140 cm) are considered by many, including most German or Japanese endoscopists, to be a good compromise, almost always reaching the cecum. The only advantage of using 70 cm flexible sigmoidoscopes for limited examinations is that the endoscopist knows from the onset that the procedure will be limited, so avoiding the temptation to go further. However, since flexible sigmoidoscopy can be performed with a longer instrument (a pediatric colonoscope is ideal) there is little need to purchase flexible sigmoidoscopes for an endoscopy unit, although they may have an essential role in the office of a primary-care physician or an out-patient clinic facility.

Variable-stiffness colonoscopes (Innoflex®, Olympus Optical Co.) have a twist control on the shaft (Fig. 6.2a) that forcibly compresses and rigidifies an internal steel coil (similar to a brake cable on a bicycle) (Fig. 6.2b,c). Compressing the coil stiffens it and also the shaft/insertion tube within which it lies. The last 30 cm to the tip of the bending section is left 'floppy' at all times. The bonus of using a variable-stiffness colonoscope is that, without having to withdraw and exchange instruments, the endoscopist can select relatively 'floppy' shaft mode to pass looping sections of the colon, then apply 'stiffer' mode to discourage re-looping when the scope has been straightened out, typically at the splenic flexure. Variable-stiffness scopes thus combine, in one colonoscope, many of the virtues of both standard and pediatric instruments. They prove significantly easier to use in most patients found previously to be 'difficult' to examine—especially where the problem was due to uncontrollable looping and discomfort. Since any first-time patient may prove to be difficult, a long variable-stiffness instrument is our 'colonoscope of choice'.

Pediatric colonoscopes, of intermediate length and smaller diameter (9–10 mm), are available with either standard, 'floppy' or variable shaft characteristics. They are invaluable for the examination of babies and children up to 2–3 years of age but also have a role to play in adult endoscopy. As well as allowing examination of strictures, anastomoses or stomas impassable with the full-sized colonoscope, they are often much easier to pass through areas of tethered postoperative adhesions or severe diverticu-

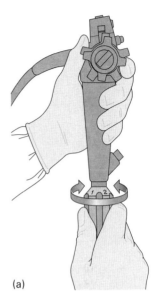

(a)

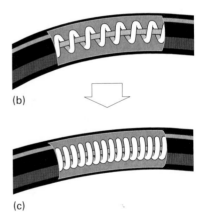

(b)

(c)

Fig. 6.2 (a) Variable-stiffness colonoscopes have a twist control on the shaft. (b) A pull-wire within an internal steel coil … (c)… compresses the coil and stiffens it (and the scope).

lar disease. The pediatric instrument bending section is more flexible, making it easier to obtain a retroverted view of some awkwardly placed polyps, whether in the distal or transverse colon, in order to ensure complete removal. Floppy pediatric instruments are also particularly comfortable and easy to insert to the splenic flexure, tending to conform to the loops of the colon and to form a spontaneous 'alpha' loop, which avoids difficulty in passing to the descending colon. The smaller diameter of the shaft is, however, less easy to torque or twist and is more easily damaged if used routinely for more extensive examination. For limited adult examinations, as for strictures or diverticular disease, a pediatric gastroscope can also be used (and has the bonus of an even shorter bending section, but the disadvantage of limited downward angling capability). Its very stiff shaft makes it less suitable for total colonoscopy in small children and babies than the pediatric colonoscope.

Accessories

All the usual accessories are used down the colonoscope, including biopsy forceps, snares, retrieval forceps or baskets, sclerotherapy needles, cytology brushes, washing catheters, dilating balloons, etc. Long- and intermediate-length accessories work equally well down shorter instruments, so it is sensible to order all accessories to suit the longest instrument in routine use. Other manufacturers' accessories also work down any particular instrument and, since some are better than others, it is worth taking advice when buying replacements. A rarely seen specialized accessory for colonoscopy is the stiffening tube, splinting device or split overtube, the use of which is described later (p. 143). Although not used by many endoscopists, and potentially hazardous if wrongly used, it is still very occasionally invaluable in avoiding recurrent loop formation of the sigmoid colon, for exchange of instruments or for retrieving multiple polyps.

Carbon dioxide

Few colonoscopists, regrettably, use CO_2 insufflation, although its use has much to commend it from the patient's point of view. CO_2 was originally used instead of air because of the explosive potential of colonic gases during electrosurgery. However, with the exception of bowel preparation using mannitol, the prepared colon has been shown to have no residual explosive gas. Nonetheless, even for routine examinations, the use of CO_2 offers the striking advantage that it is cleared from the colon 100 times faster than air (through the circulation, to the lungs and then breathed out). This means that 15–20 minutes after CO_2 insufflation the colon and small intestine are free of any gas, whereas air distension can remain and cause abdominal bloating and discomfort for many hours, especially distressing for patients with functional bowel symptoms. Colonoscopy with CO_2 insufflation can be followed immediately by barium enema or a scan (air is used for most virtual colography). In the unlikely event of perforation or gas leak (pneumoperitoneum), air under pressure would add to the hazard whereas rapidly absorbed CO_2 and a well-prepared colon should markedly reduce it. Any patient with ileus, pseudo-obstruction, stricturing, severe colitis, diverticular disease or functional bowel disorder should benefit from the added safety and comfort of using CO_2 rather than air insufflation.

In some instruments it is possible to substitute a CO_2 insufflation valve (Fig. 6.3) as a replacement for the usual air/water valve, which makes instrument handling easier than activating an alternatively sited CO_2 valve. Low-pressure, controlled-flow CO_2 delivery systems with fail-safe pressure-reducing features are available (Olympus ECR); these remove the previous objection that CO_2 insufflation exposed the patient to the potential hazard of cylinder pressure in the event of conventional flow-meter failure.

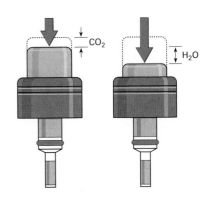

Fig. 6.3 A CO_2 valve can replace the normal air valve.

Three-dimensional (3D) magnetic imaging

There is a need to know what shaft loops have formed during colonoscope insertion and where the tip is. In 1993 two UK groups introduced prototype 3D magnetic imagers which 'position-sense' the configuration of the instrument shaft, producing a moving 3D shaded image on a computer monitor. This is achieved by means of small coils within the instrument (or in a probe passed down its instrumentation channel), which generate pulsed magnetic fields and energize larger sensor coils in a dish alongside the patient (Fig. 6.4). The system, as commercialized (Scope Guide®, Olympus), produces no stronger fields than those of a television set and is completely safe for continuous use, except for patients with cardiac pacemakers. In use 3D imaging makes many previously difficult and traumatically looping colons much easier to intubate, and also ensures that the endoscopist knows at all times where the colonoscope tip has reached and what loops may have formed. It is expected that it will rationalize many of the uncertainties of colonoscopy, and be a boon to both experts and beginners.

ANATOMY

Embryological anatomy (and 'difficult colonoscopy')

The embryology of colon development is complex and somewhat unpredictable, especially in terms of its outcome for mesenteries and fixations, which explains the extraordinarily variable configurations into which the colon can be pushed during colonoscopy.

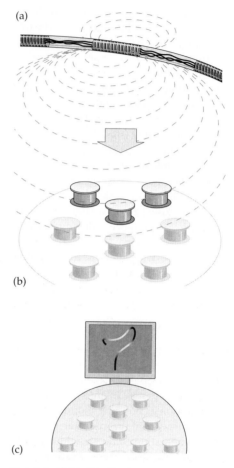

(a)

(b)

(c)

Fig. 6.4 (a) Small coils generate magnetic fields … (b)… which energize larger sensor coils in a dish alongside the patient … (c)… producing a 3D shaded image on the computer monitor.

The fetal intestine and colon initially develop as a functionless muscle tube joined at its midpoint to the yolk-stalk. This muscle tube lengthens into a U-shape on a longitudinal mesentery (Fig. 6.5a) and, as the embryo at this 5-week stage is only 1 cm long, the lengthening intestine and colon (Fig. 6.5b) are forced out into the umbilical hernia (Fig. 6.5c). The gut loop thus differentiates into the small and large intestine outside the abdominal cavity. By the third month of development the embryo is 4 cm long and there is room within the peritoneal cavity for first the small and then the large intestine to be returned into the abdomen. This occurs in a fairly predictable manner, with the end result that the colon is rotated around so that the cecum lies in the right hypochondrium and the descending colon on the left of the abdomen (Fig. 6.6a). With further elongation of the colon, the cecum normally migrates down to the right iliac fossa. At this stage, the mesentery

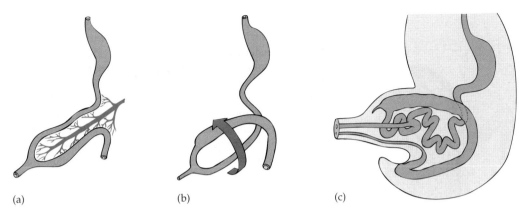

Fig. 6.5 (a) The fetal intestine and colon start on a longitudinal mesentery … (b)… then rotate as the small intestine elongates … (c)… and from 5 weeks (1 cm embryo) to 3 months (4 cm embryo) are in the umbilical hernia.

of the transverse colon is free but then the mesenteries of the descending and ascending colon, pushed against the peritoneum of the posterior abdominal wall by the fluid-filled bulky small intestine, fuse with it, so that the ascending and descending colon become retroperitoneal and fixed (Fig. 6.6b).

Incomplete fusion of the mesocolon to the posterior wall of the abdomen can therefore occur and a variable amount of the original mesocolon remains, resulting in variable mobility of the right and left colon. A mobile colon can be a nightmare for the colonoscopist because there are no fixed points at which to obtain leverage, and few of the usual 'tricks of the trade' will work, since most of them depend on withdrawal and leverage against fixations. A seductive hypothesis explaining this variation from normal development is that there is failure of enteric neuron innervation or differentiation within the intestinal muscle tube in

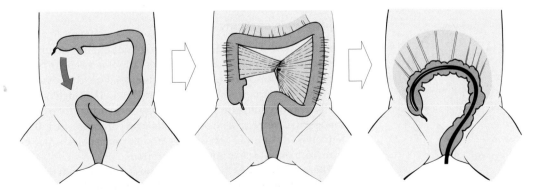

Fig. 6.6 (a) The embryonic colon extends on its mesentery at 3 months' gestation … (b)… then partial fusion of the mesentery and peritoneum occurs at 5 months … (c)… although sometimes the mesocolons persist.

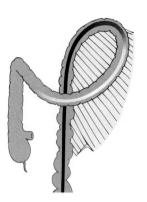

Fig. 6.7 Persistent descending mesocolon or mesentery.

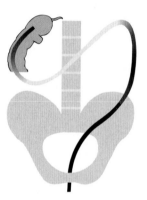

Fig. 6.8 Inverted cecum.

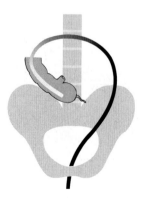

Fig. 6.9 Mobile cecum.

early embryonic development. An atonic, bulky and dysfunctional fetal intestine and colon will inevitably be retained longer than usual outside the abdomen in the umbilical hernia, until the developing abdominal cavity is large enough to reaccommodate it. Delayed return of a large colon into the abdomen means that peritoneal development will be likely to have progressed beyond the 'milestone moment' for fixation and fusion to occur (usually by 10–12 weeks after conception). The long, mobile and increasingly dysfunctional colon presents clinically at a later stage, in childhood with straining at stool and bleeding, in teenage years with constipation, or in adulthood with hemorrhoids and variable bowel habit. Endoscopically such a colon is noted to be unusually capacious, long and often atypically looping—but it can also be dramatically squashed down and shortened when the colonoscope is withdrawn at the cecum (typically to a length of only 50–60 cm), proving the lack of fixations. Further suggestive evidence that this a genetically determined constitutional abnormality of development comes from the fact that first-degree relatives (especially on the female side) are very frequently known by the patient to have disturbance of habit or constipation; if endoscoped or imaged their colons are found to be similarly long and mobile.

How often such failure of fusion, persistent colonic mesentery and mobility occurs is not clear from the literature. A persistent descending mesocolon has been found at postmortem in 36% and an ascending mesocolon in 10%. The persistence of a descending mesocolon explains most of the strange configurations caused by the colonoscope in the left colon and splenic flexure (Fig. 6.7). Occasionally the cecum fails to descend and becomes fixed in the right hypochondrium (Fig. 6.8); in others, where a free mesocolon persists, the cecum remains completely mobile (Fig. 6.9). Peroperative studies that we have undertaken show that colons in Oriental subjects are more predictably fixed than those in Western subjects.

Endoscopic anatomy

The *anal canal*, 3 cm long, extends up to the squamo–columnar junction or 'dentate line'. Sensory innervation, and hence mucosal pain sensation, may in some subjects extend up to 5–7 cm into the distal rectum. Around the canal are the anal sphincters, normally in tonic contraction. The anus may be deformed, scarred or made sensitive by present or previous local pathology, including hemorrhoids or other conditions—and normal subjects may be sore from the effects of bowel preparation.

There are two potentially serious consequences from the fact that the hemorrhoidal veins drain into the systemic (not the portal) circulation:

1 Mistakenly snaring a 'pile' can result in catastrophic hemorrhage.

2 Injecting intramucosal epinephrine (adrenaline) at a concentration greater than 1 : 200 000 before sessile polypectomy in the distal rectum has a serious risk of inducing potentially fatal cardiac or circulatory events (whereas the colonic vasculature drains via the portal system, so the liver can metabolize the higher concentrations of epinephrine often used proximally).

The *rectum*, reaching 15 cm proximal to the anal verge, may have a capacious 'ampulla' in its mid-part as well as three or more prominent partial or 'semilunar' folds (valves of Houston) that create potential blind spots, in any of which the endoscopist can miss significant pathology. Digital examination, direct inspection and, where appropriate, a rigid rectoscope/proctoscope are needed for complete examination of the area. 'Video-proctoscopy' (see below) is a convenient way of doing this. Prominent, somewhat tortuous veins are a normal feature of the rectal mucosa and should not be confused with the rare, markedly serpiginous veins of a hemangioma or the distended, tortuous ones seen in some cases of portal hypertension. The rectum is extraperitoneal for its distal 10–12 cm, making this part relatively safe for therapeutic maneuvers such as removal or destruction of sessile polyps; proximal to this it enters the abdominal cavity, invested in peritoneum.

Mucosal 'microanatomy' is visible to the discerning endoscopist. This includes the shiny surface coating of mucus, around 30% of the mucosal cells being mucus-secreting cells—described as 'goblet cells' because of their flask-shaped mucus-containing inclusions. The 'highlights' reflected off the mucus layer can show up fine underlying detail, such as the arc impressions of circular muscle fibers or the dappled, sievelike reflections caused by the microscopic crypt or pit openings. Minor abnormalities such as prominent lymphoid follicles and the smallest polyps or 'flat adenomas' often first catch the endoscopist's eye through such light reflexes off the mucus layer. The mucosal columnar epithelium, around 50 cells thick, is transparent (unlike the horny keratinized squamous epithelium of the skin surface) and through it can be seen—paired and often in exquisite detail—the venules and arterioles that make up the normal submucosal 'vascular pattern'.

The *colon musculature* develops as three external longitudinal muscle bundles, or teniae coli, and within these, the wrapping of circular muscle fibers. Both muscle layers are sometimes visible to the endoscopist (Fig. 6.10). One or more of the teniae may be seen as an inward longitudinal bulge. The circular musculature is seen as fine reflective ripples under the mucosal surface, particularly in 'spastic' or hypertonic colons. The distal colon, needing to cope with formed stools, has markedly thicker circular musculature than in the proximal colon, resulting in a tubular

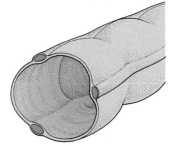

Fig. 6.10 The longitudinal muscle bundles (teniae coli) bulge visibly into the colon.

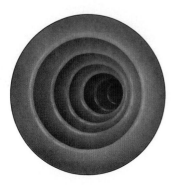

Fig. 6.11 The distal colon is usually circular.

appearance (Fig. 6.11) broken by the ridged indentations of the haustral folds.

Haustral folds segment the interior of the colon; those that are prominent in the proximal colon sometimes create 'blind spots', whereas they can be hypertrophied in sigmoid diverticular disease, creating mechanical difficulties for the endoscopist.

The three external teniae coli, or longitudinal muscle bundles, are only seen distally if the colon is abnormally capacious, bulging outwards between them. In elderly subjects the sigmoid colon anatomy is often narrowed and deformed internally by the thickened circular muscle rings of hypertrophic diverticular disease, and sometimes also fixed externally by pericolic post-inflammatory processes. Redundant and prolapsing mucosal folds overlying the muscular rings in diverticular disease often appear reddened from traumatization, and sometimes focally inflamed as well.

External structures can be seen through the colonic wall, typically as the blue-gray discoloration of the spleen or liver proximally. Vascular pulsations of the adjacent left iliac artery are often visible in the sigmoid, and right iliac artery pulsations are occasionally visible proximally. Small intestinal gas distension and peristaltic activity may be seen through the colon wall, especially at the cecal pole.

INSERTION

Pre-procedure checks should be made on all functions of the endoscope, light source and accessories before insertion. In particular make sure that air (or CO_2) insufflation is fully operational, with no rinse water remaining in the air channel. The tip should bubble briskly when held underwater (if in doubt wrap a rubber glove around the tip and watch it inflate under pressure). It is difficult to spot suboptimal insufflation (see p. 167) once the scope is inserted, and easy to think the colon is hypercontractile—when in fact one of the connections is loose, the insufflation valve or an O-ring is misplaced or faulty, or the air outlet is semi-obstructed. Any of these faults will result in decreased pressure and so only partial insufflation pressure. A clean lens and correct color (white balance of the CCD) are also important.

Inserting through the anus should be gentle. The instrument tip is unavoidably blunt (the lenses mean that it cannot be streamlined), so too fast or forcible an insertion may be painful for patients with tight sphincters or sore anal epithelium; the squamous epithelium of the anus and the sensory mechanisms of the anal sphincters are the most pain-sensitive areas in the colorectum. The patient lies in the left lateral position and the endoscopist dons examination gloves.

There are several ways of inserting the scope:

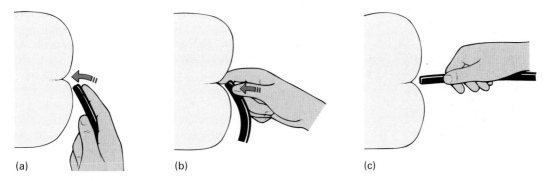

Fig. 6.12 Different methods of colonoscope insertion: (a) finger support of the bending section; (b) the tip pushed in as the examining finger withdraws; or (c) straight on through the jelly.

1 Many endoscopists start with two gloves on the right hand and perform a digital examination with a generous amount of lubricant before inserting the instrument, both to check for pathology in this potentially 'blind' area and to prelubricate and relax the anal canal. The instrument tip is passed in pressed in obliquely, supported by the examiner's forefinger until the sphincter relaxes (Fig. 6.12a).

2 Alternatively, the examiner can use the thumb to push the tip inward along the examining forefinger as this withdraws from the anal canal (Fig. 6.12b). The tendency of the bending section to flex can be avoided by starting with it straight, fixing the angulation control brakes and pressing in gently.

3 Alternatively, a large blob of lubricant jelly can be squeezed out over the anal orifice and the instrument inserted directly through it (Fig. 6.12c), which saves a glove and a few seconds. Inflating air down the endoscope while pressing the tip into the anal canal gives direct vision and facilitates insertion.

Tight or tonic sphincters may take some time to relax; asking the patient to 'bear down' is said to help this. Allowing an extra 15–20 seconds for sphincter relaxation can be a humane start to proceedings, especially for a patient with anorectal pathology or anismus—the sphincters of colitis patients are noticeably more tonic than normal, presumably because of the longstanding need to keep control.

Video-proctoscopy

Rigid proctoscopy has an important role in inspecting the anorectal area for mucosal prolapse, hemorrhoids or other pathology. The patient can be shown the appearances by the simple expedient of inserting the video-endoscope tip up the proctoscope once the insertion trocar is removed. The colonoscope simultaneously provides a convenient source of illumination and an excellent close-up view. The endoscopist can perform video-proctoscopy

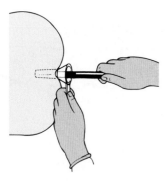

Fig. 6.13 Video-proctoscopy.

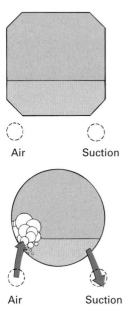

Air Suction

Air Suction

Fig. 6.14 The suction/instrumentation port opens below and to the right of the view; the air port opens below and left.

(Fig. 6.13) entirely from the monitor view, with the opportunity for taking a videotaped or printed record—which in many cases of 'unexplained bleeding' persuasively shows the patient and referring doctor the likely (hemorrhoidal) origin.

Rectal insertion

A 'red-out' is often the first view after the scope has been inserted into the rectum. This is because the lens is pressed against the rectal mucosa. The following steps should be performed, in sequence:

1 Insufflate air to distend the rectum.

2 Pull back and angulate or rotate slightly to find the lumen (this is the first of many times during the examination when withdrawal, inspection and cerebration bring success more quickly than following instinct and pushing blindly).

3 Rotate the view so that any fluid lies inferiorly. The suction port of the colonoscope tip lies just below the bottom righthand corner of the image (Fig. 6.14) and should be selectively placed in the fluid before activating the suction valve. To do this coordination will be required between active shaft rotation with the right hand and synchronous compensatory up or down angulation with the left hand so as to keep the view. During examination a skilled single-handed endoscopist often uses twist to torque-steer or 'corkscrew' the tip; the capacious rectum is the ideal place in which to practice this, using the need to suction fluid as a good excuse to do so.

4 Aspirate fluid or residue to avoid any chance of anorectal leakage during the rest of the examination. The warm, lubricated colonoscope shaft moving in and out often gives the patient a distressing illusion of being incontinent. Knowing that there is no rectal fluid to leak out and that any gas can be released without fear of an accident is much appreciated.

5 Push in, finally, only when an adequate view has been obtained, and only as fast as a reasonable view can be obtained.

6 Torque-steer round the first few bends, using up or down angulation and shaft-twist alone to achieve most lateral movements, rather than unnecessarily using the lateral angulation control. This is an economic way of steering in at this stage and demonstrates the efficacy of finger twist when the shaft is straight—which it inevitably is in the recto-sigmoid region.

Retroversion

Retroversion can be important in the rectum because the latter, often being very capacious, can be surprisingly difficult to examine completely. Care is needed to combine angling and twist movements sufficiently to see behind the major folds or valves. In a capacious rectum the most distal part is a potential blind spot, but the generous size of the rectal ampulla will usually make tip retroflexion relatively easy. Choose the widest part, angulate both controls fully and push gently inward to invert the tip toward the anal verge (Fig. 6.15). Retroversion is *not* always possible in a small or narrowed rectum, but in a narrow rectum the wide-angled (140°, nearly 'fish-eye') lens of the endoscope should see everything without risk of blind spots.

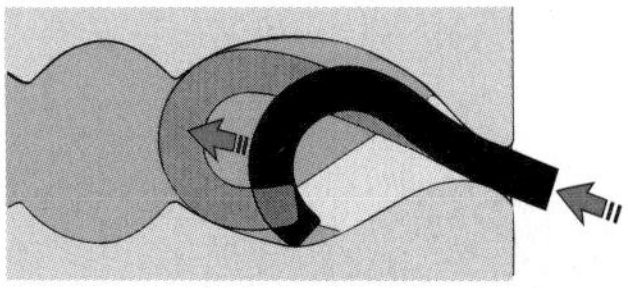

Fig. 6.15 Angulate both valves and *push in* to retrovert.

HANDLING—'SINGLE-HANDED', 'TWO-HANDED' OR TWO-PERSON?

Most skilled endoscopists favor the one-person 'single-handed' approach in which the colonoscopist manages all controls with one hand and the shaft with the other. But there are many who use two hands on the angulation controls and a few experts who work successfully with the 'two-person' method, using an assistant to manipulate the shaft. This situation arises from the fact that all current endoscopes originate from gastroscope design, where the shorter, straighter gastric anatomy and the stiffer insertion tube make 'two-hand' management of the up/down and lateral angulation controls more logical. Flexible sigmoidoscopy, especially if using a 70 cm instrument, perhaps also lends itself to this handling approach.

'Single-handed' one-person colonoscopy

In 'single-handed' colonoscopy the endoscopist manages the colonoscope controls with the left hand, leaving the right hand free to hold the shaft (Fig. 6.16). This gives the endoscopist com-

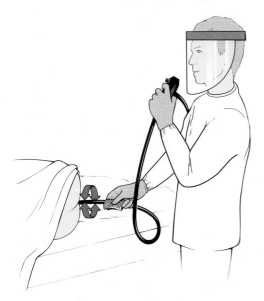

Fig. 6.16 Single-handed maneuvering of the instrument shaft.

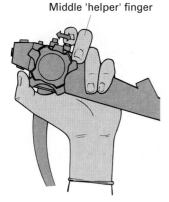

Middle 'helper' finger

Fig. 6.17 Single-handed control: the forefinger alone activates the air/water and suction valves; the middle finger acts as 'helper' to the thumb for angulation.

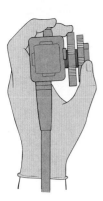

Fig. 6.18 The thumb can reach the lateral angulation control if the hand is positioned appropriately.

plete control and the opportunity at all times to *feel* the colonoscope interacting with loops and bends.

The endoscopist should grip the shaft (insertion tube) 25–30 cm away from the anus. Many people make the mistake of holding too close to the anus, resulting in the need for frequent changes of hand-grip and jerky insertion technique. Holding the shaft further back makes for smoother insertion, easier application of torque (maintained twisting force) and better feel of the forces involved.

Handling efficiency can be increased by disciplining the fingers of the left hand (Fig. 6.17). Using only *two* fingers, the fourth (ring finger) and the little finger, to grip the control body lets the middle finger assume an invaluable 'helper' role to the thumb. Most endoscopists, unthinkingly but unnecessarily, use three fingers to hold the control body—and then wonder why angulation can be so awkward. Single-handed steering is also made easier if the first finger alone operates the air/water or suction valves, again so as to leave the middle finger free to act as 'helper' to the thumb in managing the angulation controls. For those with reasonably large hands it is practicable for the left thumb to reach both the up/down and the lateral angulation controls (Fig. 6.18).

Right-hand 'torque steering' twisting the shaft at the same time as angulating the tip up or down, is how the skilled single-handed colonoscopist achieves most lateral movements, rather than using the lateral angulation control too often. The right hand can also feel whether the shaft moves easily (is straight) or there is resistance (due to looping). To be able to feel and manipulate the shaft deftly, hold it in the fingers (Fig. 6.19) as you would with any other delicate instrument, such as a small electrical screwdriver, and not in the fist—like a hammer or an offensive weapon. Rolling the shaft between fingers and thumb allows major steering rotations of up to 360°—whereas wrist-twist manages only 180°.

'Two-handed' one-person technique

The 'two-handed technique' is mainly used by those with small hands, who may be unable to reach the lateral angulation control with the left thumb and so may need, from time to time, to use the right hand for this purpose. This unfortunately means briefly letting go of the instrument shaft while the angulation is made. Some endoscopists position the patient so that they can lean and trap the colonoscope shaft transiently against the couch while the right hand is otherwise occupied. If the right hand is used too often for lateral steering it is likely that the endoscopist is not torque-steering efficiently. Equally, if the right hand is away from the shaft for too long in order to work the lateral angulation control, the endoscopist is being indecisive—it takes at most a second or two to make the angulation control adjustment and then return the hand to shaft management.

Two-person colonoscopy

Two-person colonoscopy relies on an assistant to handle the shaft. This allows the endoscopist to use the control body of the instrument in the way that it is (unfortunately) currently designed—namely with the left hand working the up/down control and air/water/suction valves and the right hand adjusting the right/left angulation control. The assistant performs the role ascribed to the right hand of the single-handed endoscopist, pushing and pulling according to the spoken instructions of the endoscopist. A good assistant learns to feel the shaft to some extent and to apply some twist. More often, the assistant pushes with concealed gusto, causing unnecessary loops that are not apparent to the endoscopist but painful for the patient. Unless endoscopist/assistant teamwork is skilled and interactive, the two-person approach to colonoscopy can be as illogical and clumsy as would be expected of two people attempting any other intricate task, neither quite knowing what the other is doing. In occasional difficult situations, for instance passing an awkward angulation or snaring a difficult polyp, all endoscopists justifiably use the assistant briefly to control the shaft for a moment or two.

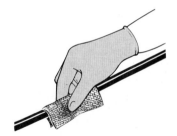

Fig. 6.19 The instrument shaft should be held delicately between the thumb and fingers.

SINGLE-HANDED STEERING

Stance should be relaxed and the endoscopist should also hold the colonoscope in a relaxed manner. Colonoscopy mostly requires fine and fluent movements, like those of a violin player—a similarly balanced position and handling are needed. The modification of endoscopist stance and patient position used by some 'two-handed' endoscopists has been mentioned above, the patient being positioned close to the edge of the trolley or cart so that the shaft can hang down, allowing the single-handed endoscopist to trap it with thigh pressure from time to time.

Logical steering responses depend on quick, almost reflex, coordination between the right and left hands, which comes with practice. Colonoscopy, from slow deliberate beginnings, can become a relatively rapid and fluent procedure.

Key points for colonoscope steering are as follows:
- Twisting (torquing) the shaft only affects the tip when the shaft is straight (Fig. 6.20). When a loop is present in the shaft, twisting forces applied will be lost within the loop. When the shaft is straight, twist becomes an excellent way to torque or

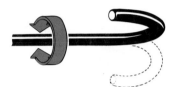

Fig. 6.20 Twist only affects the tip if the shaft is straight.

corkscrew around bends. This is particularly useful if the angle to be traversed is acute or fixed, because simply trying to push around will encounter severe resistance (often resulting in looping rather than progress).

• Torque steering involves first angulating up or down as appropriate and, rather than using the lateral angulation control, torquing (twisting, rotating) the instrument shaft clockwise or counterclockwise with the right hand. Because the tip is already slightly angled this rotation should corkscrew it around laterally (Fig. 6.21), precisely and quickly, and will often make use of the lateral angulation control unnecessary. Torquing is also a valuable way of orienting the scope tip and bending section in order to target lesions accurately, making biopsy-taking or polypectomy quicker and easier. Torque steering is, inevitably, affected by the direction in which the tip is angulated, With 'up-angulation', clockwise torque moves the tip to the right, whereas it moves to the *left* if angulation is down.

• When torque (maintained twist) is used to control a loop, steering may have to be with the angulation controls. The principles of loop control are discussed below, but strong twisting movements are a key. It is essential to realize that if, in order to steer, the torque applied to hold a loop straight has to be released, the loop will re-form. Maintaining the shaft torque but applying the relevant angulating control avoids this.

• Steering with the lateral angulation control has least effect when the tip is already maximally angled (up or down). Try this outside the patient. When one control is fully angulated, applying the other one swivels the bending section a little but hardly affects the degree of angulation (Fig. 6.22). Vicious steering movements are therefore rarely helpful (and can damage the angulation control wires).

• A fully angulated tip will not slide along the colon. It is easy to forget, in the quest to get a view around bends, that overan-

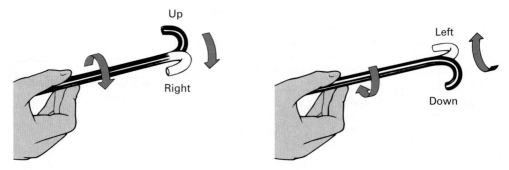

Fig. 6.21 With a clockwise shaft twist: (a) an up-angled tip moves to the right … (b)… and a down-angled tip moves to the left.

gulation can be counterproductive (the 'walking-stick handle' phenomenon) (Fig. 6.23).

• An impacted tip cannot be steered. The bending section of flexible endoscopes normally angulates because it is free to move, and the shaft is relatively stiffer and more fixed. If the tip of the bending section is fixed, on attempted angulation the shaft moves instead. Try it yourself (outside the patient). Hold the tip of the bending section very firmly and operate the angulation control(s). The shaft will move because the tip cannot (Fig. 6.24). This is an inherent limiting factor of flexible endoscopes, and is why the endoscopist is sometimes so impotent in fixed diverticular disease or a tight stricture. Torque is less affected in such situations—another reason why torque-steering is so useful in colonoscopy.

• Use the lateral angulation control as little as possible. There are a limited number of possible tip-steering movements for the single-handed endoscopist:

(a) the easiest is up/down thumb control (left hand);

(b) the next easiest is clockwise/counterclockwise twist (right hand);

(c) the least convenient is left/right angulation (either by the left thumb or the right hand).

• Coordinate left and right hand activities. The endoscopist is like a puppeteer propelling a snake puppet by the tail, with control of its head, a view through its eyes, but scant idea of what is happening to the snake body—because this is invisible within the abdomen. For single-handed endoscopy, in order to control the snake fluently and efficiently, each hand must be disciplined to fulfill only its appropriate tasks. The left hand holds the instrument in balance, manages the air/water/suction valves and up/down angulation control (Fig. 6.16), adding minor thumb adjustments of left/right angulation when needed (Fig. 6.18). Because the colon is a continuous series of short bends, requiring multiple combinations of tip angulation and shaft movement and frequent air/water and suction valve activations, small delays

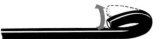

Fig. 6.22 The lateral control angulation has little effect if the tip is maximally up/down-angled.

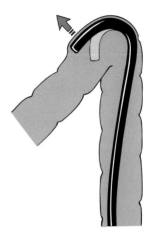

Fig. 6.23 De-angulate at the splenic flexure to avoid impaction—the 'walking-stick handle' effect.

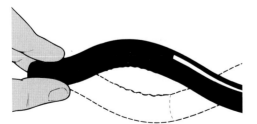

Fig. 6.24 If the tip is fixed it cannot be steered (the shaft moves instead).

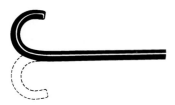

Fig. 6.25 A single-handed dexterity test: five full up/down angulations can be done in 20 seconds.

and uncoordinated movements rapidly summate, prolonging the procedure unnecessarily.

A table-top dexterity test will check efficiency of left-hand angulation technique, or will at least demonstrate the problems. Perform five full bending section retroflexions from maximally up to maximally down (with no help from the right hand); this can be done in around 20 seconds—but only fully and rapidly (and single-handedly) if the 'helper finger' is brought into action (Figs 6.17 and 6.25).

Insertion through the colon should be as quick as reasonably possible because the pushing and looping of the insertion phase is uncomfortable and stressful for the patient. Full inspection should be on the return journey—although better views of some areas are obtained on the way in when the colon is stretched; any small polyps seen should therefore be destroyed during the insertion phase, because they can easily be missed in the shortened colon on the way back. However, trying to hurry colonoscope insertion, using aggression and force to attempt speed, is usually self-defeating and ends up in a slower, traumatic or failed insertion. The sigmoid colon is an elastic tube (Fig. 6.26). Inflated it becomes long and tortuous; deflated it is significantly shorter. When stretched by a colonoscope, especially if overinflated as well, the bowel forms loops and acute bends (Fig. 6.27) but if shortened down and deflated it can be telescoped into a few convoluted centimeters (Fig. 6.28) (rather like pushing a coat- or shirt-sleeve up to expose the arm).

The following are simple general principles for comfortable and safe insertion:

• *Suction air frequently and fluid infrequently*. A perfect view isn't necessary during insertion. Whenever fully distended colon is seen or if the patient feels discomfort it takes only a second or two

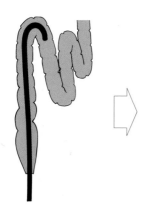

Fig. 6.26 The sigmoid colon is an elastic tube …

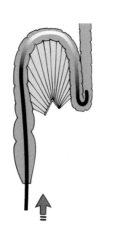

Fig. 6.27 … pushing loops it …

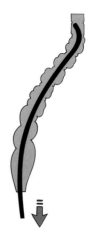

Fig. 6.28 … but pulling back shortens and straightens the colon.

to suction off excess air until the colon outline starts to wrinkle and collapse, making it shorter and also easier to manipulate. In contrast, after having evacuated fluid from the rectum, only aspirate fluid during the rest of the insertion phase when absolutely necessary to keep a view, and only do so when there is enough air present and a good enough view to suction accurately (sucking blind when already immersed is usually rather ineffectual). During insertion there will be numerous local 'sumps' or pools of residual fluid; aspirating each one wastes a lot of time, loses the view and requires reinflation. It is usually possible to inflate a little and steer in over the fluid level rather than plunging into it and having to suction. Even solid stool can often be successfully passed, deliberately angling the tip to slide along the mucosa for a few centimeters rather than impacting against a bolus, which can coat the lens irrevocably. Any residue can easily be suctioned or removed from view by changes of patient position on the way back when a perfect view is important.

• *Insufflate as little as possible.* A distended colon is less manageable and more uncomfortable. Gentle insufflation *is* needed throughout the examination to keep a view. However, the policy is 'as much as necessary, as little as possible'; it is essential to see, but counterproductive to overinflate. Remember that bubbles are caused by insufflating under water (Fig. 6.14), which can usually be avoided by the simple means of angling above it. If fluid preparation and bile salts do result in excessive bubbles, these can be dispersed instantly by injecting an antifoam preparation solution containing particulate silicone down the instrument channel.

• *Use all visual clues.* A perfect view is not needed for progress; but the correct direction or axis of the colonic lumen should be ascertained *before* pushing in. The lumen when deflated or in spasm is at the center of converging folds (Fig. 6.29). With only a partial or close-up view of the mucosal surface, there are usually sufficient clues to detect the luminal direction. Aim toward the darkest (worst illuminated) area because it is furthest from the instrument and nearest the lumen (Fig. 6.30). The convex arcs formed by visible wrinkling of the circular muscles, or the haustral folds or the highlights reflected from the mucosa over them, indicate the center of the arc as the correct direction in which to angle (Fig. 6.31). The slight bulge of the underlying longitudinal muscle bundles (teniae coli) is another, occasionally useful, clue. The expert can make his steering decisions on evidence that would be inadequate for the beginner. On the other hand, each time the expert is 'lost' for more than 5–10 seconds he pulls back quickly to regain the view and reorientate, whereas the beginner can flounder around blindly for a minute or more in each difficult spot and is surprised that the overall examination takes so long.

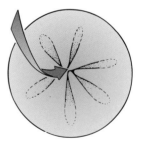

Fig. 6.29 Aim at the convergence of folds.

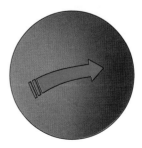

Fig. 6.30 Aim at the darkest area.

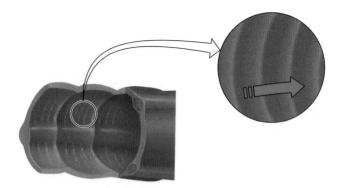

Fig. 6.31 Aim at the center of the arc formed by folds, muscle fibers or reflected highlights.

• *Steer carefully and cautiously.* Steering movements should be early, slow and exact (rather than jerky and erratic). A slow start to each angulation movement allows it to be terminated at once, within a few degrees of travel, if it proves to be moving the tip in the wrong direction. A rapid steering movement in the wrong direction can simply lose the view altogether, quite unnecessarily, and then tends to be corrected by another large movement so that the effect is to flail around—often hopelessly, and certainly inelegantly. Each individual movement should be slow and purposive, and every action during insertion should be thought out and executed in response to the view, or whatever visual clues there are to suggest the correct luminal direction. Don't thrash around with the scope tip—look and think instead.

• *Rehearse steering actions* before bends while there is a good view. Unlike the stomach, where there is usually sufficient room to see what is happening during steering maneuvers, colonic bends are unforgivingly tight and it is very easy to become unsighted and uncertain when angling around them. Stop before any acute bend and try out, while stationary and still able to see, the best steering movements to use within it.

• *'Set up' bends* so that steering around the axis is easier. During upper gastrointestinal endoscopy, the instrument is ideally made to run around the axis of the greater curve to reach the antrum and pylorus (see Fig. 4.15). Similarly, the colonoscopist should, whenever possible, adjust the instrument so that an acute bend can be passed with its axis upward or downward (for easy thumb steering), as well as optimizing mechanical efficiency by having the colonoscope shaft straight (for better push) and the bending section not overangled (to help it slide around). A good 'racing line' is fundamental to ski and car racing and, at infinitely slower speed, is just as applicable to non-traumatic flexible endoscopy.

- *If there is no view, pull back at once.* Pushing blindly, especially if there is a 'red-out' and total loss of view, is usually a pointless waste of time, and potentially a cause of perforation. If lost at any point in the examination, keep the angulation controls still or let them go entirely, insufflate and then gently withdraw the instrument until the mucosa and its vascular pattern slips slowly past the lens in a proximal direction (Fig. 6.32); follow the direction of slippage by angulating the controls or twisting the shaft, and the lumen of the colon will come back into view. Thrashing around blindly with the instrument rarely works; *pulling back* must do, for the bending section self-straightens if left free to do so.

- *Think of position change if the view is poor,* especially due to excess fluid. Especially if the patient can co-operate, repositioning should save much more time than it takes for the patient to change from left lateral to supine or right lateral, letting gravity repasture fluid and gas (and the colon also—often beneficially).

- *Keep the scope as straight as possible.* Every endoscopist knows the benefits of straightening back a gastroscope in allowing easier maneuvering in the duodenum (see Fig. 4.20). The meanderings and looping tendency of the colon makes this principle even more critical during colonoscopy. Mechanically too, if inward shaft push is to be transmitted to the tip and the scope is to work with maximal efficiency, it must be kept as straight as possible. The mechanical construction of an endoscope, with its protective wire claddings and four angulation wires, means that each shaft loop increases the resistance of the instrument to twisting/torquing movements, and decreases tip angulation by causing friction in the angulation wires. For this reason shaft loops are also as counterproductive *outside* the patient as inside the abdomen. Thus the shaft should be made to run in an easy curve to the anus, without unnecessary bends, and any loops forming outside the patient should be derotated and straightened. This is best done by rotating the control body to transfer the loop to the umbilical, which can accommodate up to three to four loops without harm to its internal structures (Fig. 6.33). Where possible the shaft of the long colonoscope should be arranged on the table so as to make it easy to twist clockwise, since this is such a frequent action.

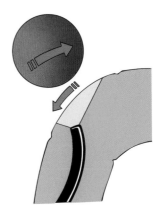

Fig. 6.32 Pull back when lost—the mucosa slides away in the direction of the lumen.

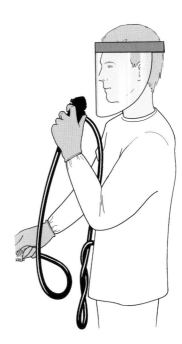

Fig. 6.33 Shaft loops forming *outside* the patient can be transferred to the umbilical by rotating the control body.

SIGMOID LOOPS

Endoscopic anatomy

The sigmoid colon is 40–70 cm long when stretched by the instrument during insertion, although it will crumple down to only 30–35 cm when the instrument is straightened fully—which is why careful inspection is important during insertion if lesions are not to be missed during the withdrawal phase. The sigmoid colon mesentery is inserted in a V-shape across the pelvic brim,

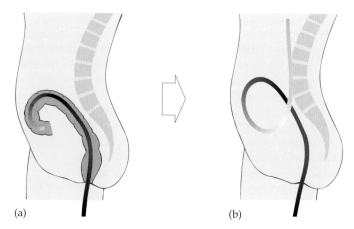

Fig. 6.34 (a) The sigmoid colon loops anteriorly … (b) … then passes up into the left paravertebral gutter.

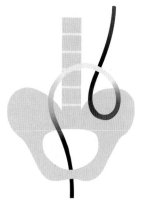

Fig. 6.35 Sigmoid loop—anterior view (clockwise spiral).

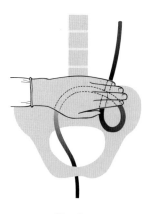

Fig. 6.36 Hand pressure restricts the sigmoid spiral loop.

but is very variable in both insertion and length, and also quite frequently modified by adhesions from previous inflammatory disease or surgery. After hysterectomy the distal sigmoid colon can be angulated and fixed anteriorly into the space vacated by the uterus.

The inserted colonoscope may stretch the bowel to the limits of its attachments or the confines of the abdominal cavity. The shape of the pelvis, with curved sacral hollow and the forward-projecting sacral promontory, cause the colonoscope to pass anteriorly (Fig. 6.34a) so that the shaft can often be felt looped onto the anterior abdominal wall before it passes posteriorly again to the descending colon in the left paravertebral gutter (Fig. 6.34b). The result is that an anteroposterior loop occurs during passage of the sigmoid colon and, since the descending colon is usually laterally placed, it forms a clockwise spiral loop (Fig. 6.35); the importance of this will be discussed later (see pp. 129–132). When the sigmoid loop runs anteriorly against the abdominal wall it is possible partially to reduce or modify the sigmoid looping of the colonoscope by pressing against the left lower abdomen with the hand (Fig. 6.36).

The descending colon is normally bound down retroperitoneally and ideally runs in a fixed straight line, which is easy to pass with the colonoscope, except that there is usually an acute bend at the junction with the sigmoid colon (Fig. 6.37). This junction is only a theoretical landmark to the radiologist but, once the sigmoid colon is deformed upwards by the inserted colonoscope shaft, the resulting angulation becomes a very real challenge to the endoscopist. The acuteness of the sigmoid-descending angle depends on anatomical factors, including how far down in the pelvis the descending colon is fixed, but also on colonoscopic insertion technique. A really acute hairpin bend results when

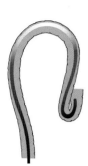

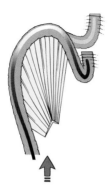

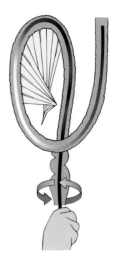

Fig. 6.37 Fixed (iatrogenic) hair-pin bend at the sigmoid–descending colon junction.

Fig. 6.38 The length of mesentery and the extent of retroperitoneal fixation determine the acuteness of the sigmoid–descending colon junction.

Fig. 6.39 An alpha loop—a beneficial iatrogenic volvulus.

the sigmoid colon is long or elastic enough to make a large loop, and the retroperitoneal fixation of the descending colon happens also to be low in the pelvis (Fig. 6.38). Sometimes, when the sigmoid colon is long an alpha loop occurs, which, blessedly for both endoscopist and patient, avoids any angulation at the sigmoid–descending junction. The 'alpha' describes the shape of the spiral loop of sigmoid colon twisted around on its mesentery or sigmoid mesocolon into a partial iatrogenic volvulus (Fig. 6.39). Formation of the loop depends on the anatomical fact that the short inverted 'V' base of the sigmoid mesocolon twists easily—providing that the sigmoid is long enough and that there are no adhesions.

Mesenteric fixation variations occur in at least 15% of subjects because of partial or complete failure of retroperitoneal fixation of the descending colon *in utero* (see p. 109). The result is persistence of varying degrees of descending mesocolon, which in turn has a considerable effect on what shapes the colonoscope can push the colon into during insertion; the descending colon can, for instance, run up the midline (Fig. 6.40) or allow a 'reversed alpha' loop to form (Fig. 6.41). Surgeons are well aware that there is great patient-to-patient variation in how easily the colon can be mobilized and delivered outside the abdominal cavity; occasionally the whole colon can be lifted out without dissection. A colon that is 'easy' for the surgeon to mobilize is, however, often extremely unpredictable and difficult for the endoscopist.

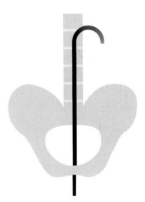

Fig. 6.40 The endoscope may push a fully mobile distal colon up the midline.

Recognizing loop formation

Recognizing that a loop is forming doesn't take genius, but it's surprising how many endoscopists 'push on regardless' on the

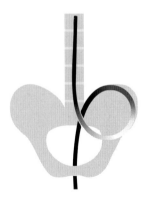

Fig. 6.41 A reversed alpha loop due to a persistent descending mesocolon.

basis that 'the view is good'—in spite of the protests of the patient. Pain is the commonest warning of loop formation, but it is more subtle to recognize a loop from *loss of 'one-to-one' relationship* between the amount of shaft being inserted and inward progress of the scope tip. *'Paradoxical movement,'* the instrument apparently sliding out as the shaft is pushed in (or vice versa), indicates that there is a substantial loop.

There may be more than one loop, resulting in the instrument feeling 'jammed up'. As the shaft loops more and more it becomes progressively less responsive to manipulation. Because of the increasing friction in the wires leading down to the bending section, the angulation controls also feel stiffer and stiffer—but have less and less effect. The difficulty is that inexperienced and tense endoscopists don't notice this and all too easily become deaf to protest, overgenerous with sedation and liable to think that forceful management of the colonoscope is 'normal'. It is important to be aware that colonoscopy can be a deft and gentle procedure, to expect to hold and feel the instrument in the *fingers* (Fig. 6.19), and to be aware that most loops can (and should) be as rapidly removed as they have formed.

Avoiding or minimizing sigmoid loops

Sigmoid looping of some degree is unavoidable as the scope pushes toward the apex of the sigmoid colon. It helps to warn the patient when 'stretch pain' will be felt, and to try to keep this to 20–30 seconds. In this time the scope should slide around the whole of a short sigmoid loop but, in longer colons, pull back to give the patient relief and to try to reduce whatever loop has started to form. It may be worth pointing out that the typical sigmoid colon is entirely passive, tortuous perhaps and subject to gravity. It is the force of colonoscope insertion that creates loops, and the challenge to the colonoscopist is to minimize or modify looping in any way that makes insertion easier.

Abdominal hand-pressure often helps a little during sigmoid insertion, since the sigmoid loop frequently loops anteriorly close to the abdominal wall (see Fig. 6.34)—especially in those with a protuberant abdomen. The assistant compresses non-specifically over the lower abdomen, which opposes the sigmoid loop, may reduce stretch pain and can make the scope slide around more easily because the loop is made smaller. Assistant hand pressure is only relevant during the (?20–30 seconds or so) needed for inward scope-push. There is no need to fatigue the assistant by asking for more prolonged hand pressure, especially as in around 50% of patients the sigmoid loop is *not* near the abdominal surface.

Push little and slowly; pull often and fast. The challenge in a longer and tortuous sigmoid is to progress the instrument tip through without repeatedly losing the view, minimizing colon and colonoscope looping as far as possible. Pushing movements should therefore start slowly, giving time for accurate torque-steering movements and allowing the endoscope to slide in (rather than just buckle upwards, as tends to happen with a rapid push). By contrast, the withdrawal movements needed to straighten out loops in the shaft and colon must be vigorous to be fully effective. An inexperienced endoscopist tends to be overcautious in pulling back. An expert starts withdrawal movements quickly and only slows down pull-back when the tip starts to slip back excessively, the shaft feels straighter and more responsive or there is the 'catapult' feel of pulling against the hooked tip. As the shaft straightens and the loop reduces, applying shaft torque may start to help (clockwise or counterclockwise, whichever seems to be more effective).

Navigating through the sigmoid colon

Torque-steering, single-handedly, is particularly useful in passing the multiple bends of the sigmoid, where coordination with an assistant can be difficult. Each of the succession of serpentine bends requires a conscious steering decision. It is easier to judge direction around a bend from afar, so the tip should not be rushed into it. First observe the bend carefully from a distance; it will be seen as a bright semilunar fold of mucosa against the shadowed background (Fig. 6.42). Having decided on the direction to be taken, try out in mini-movement rehearsal (a few millimeters or degrees of movement are enough) the best combination of angling and rotation needed to steer around correctly when subsequently pushing through the bend, often close-up and relatively blind. If finger rotation of the shaft is used much of the sigmoid can be traversed with little or no use of the lateral angulation control, the angled tip corkscrewing first one way and then the other round the succession of bends.

Acute and mobile bends are a particular problem in the sigmoid. Having angled around an acute bend, if the view is poor gently pull back the angled/hooked tip, which should simultaneously reduce the angle, shorten the bowel distally, straighten it out proximally and disimpact the tip to improve the view (Fig. 6.43). If necessary, de-angle, pull back below the bend again and recheck its direction more carefully. The colon can rotate on its attachments and the nature of bends may change during maneuvering, any rotation being visible in close-up as a rotation of the visible vessel pattern (Fig. 6.44). Watch the vessel pattern rotation carefully in close-up to know which direction to follow in a mobile bend.

Concentration is vital. Obsessional attention to keeping the endoscopic view at all times is a key aspect of efficient and accurate colonoscopy. In order not to lose orientation or miss diagnostic minutiae, the endoscopist must learn to suppress normal social reflexes—such as looking at the patient or endoscopy room staff

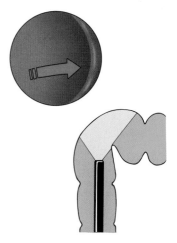

Fig. 6.42 Endoscopic view of an acute bend, with a bright fold on the angle, and the 'aerial' view.

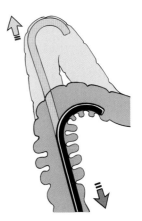

Fig. 6.43 Pulling back flattens out an acute bend and improves the view.

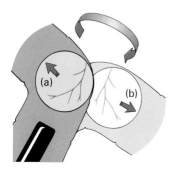

Fig. 6.44 Rotation of the vessel pattern (from (a) to (b)) indicates rotation of the colon, so the endoscopist needs to change the steering direction.

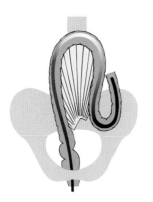

Fig. 6.45 A very long sigmoid may allow the scope to loop enough to avoid a hairpin bend.

when talking to them—in order to concentrate on the monitor view. It is perfectly possible to hold a conversation or to give instructions without eye contact, and it can be very important to do so. Some acute bends or small polyps, for instance, may slip from view in the moment that the endoscopist looks away, and then take a surprising time to find again. Intense concentration, on both mechanical and visual aspects of the procedure, makes colonoscopy quicker and more efficient. It takes all the endoscopist's faculties to assess the view, predict the correct action, keep a running mental log of decisions taken and their result, while constantly optimizing the situation or reversing ineffective actions rapidly when necessary. Colonoscopy is an algorithm of small responses to ever-varying situations. It takes a surprising degree of alertness, motivation and concentration to do it efficiently.

Push-through

Gentle 'push through' the sigmoid colon, using careful steering combined with 'persuasive pressure' may sometimes allow the scope to slide successfully around the bends of the sigmoid and up into the descending colon. This typically occurs in long colons with longer, more mobile, mesenteries which allow the instrument to loop upwards but then adapt to allow passage into the descending colon without the acute hairpin bend usually formed by N-loop stretch (Fig. 6.45). Paradoxically, shorter sigmoid loops tend to require more subtlety and cause more pain, since their shorter mesenteric attachments are more aggressively stretched.

Pain on passing the sigmoid colon indicates looping and potential danger of damage to the bowel or mesentery. Having to use force or cause pain is inelegant as well as potentially dangerous, and should be avoided as far as possible. Before using force, and at any stage during colonoscopy when pushing in may cause pain due to looping, the patient is warned beforehand (e.g. 'this will hurt for a few seconds, but there is no danger'). Inward push should also be applied gradually, avoiding any sudden shoves and should be limited to a tolerable time—no more than 20–30 seconds. Looping pain stops at once when the instrument is withdrawn slightly. There is no excuse for long continued periods of pain, even in those miserable examinations when recurrent looping cannot be avoided. However, as a last resort, it may very occasionally be preferable for the endoscopist to persuade the instrument into the descending colon quickly and successfully, rather than to struggle on with repeated failed attempts at gentle passage. Stretch pain is distressing for the patient and the analgesic effects of intravenous medication diminish considerably by about 5 minutes after administration.

Blind 'slide-by' of the instrument tip is permissable from time to time, but only if unavoidable and for a few seconds. Providing the tip is angulated correctly into the axis of an acute bend, the scope should slip gradually over the surface with the 'slide-by' appearance of mucosal vascular pattern traversing the field of view. Only push if 'slide-by' continues smoothly. Stop pushing and pull back to re-find the view after 5–10 seconds. Stop *immediately* if the mucosa blanches (indicating excessive local pressure) or if the patient experiences pain (indicating undue strain on the bowel or mesentery). This is the moment that precedes perforation—and so the moment to change tack, change position, change endoscopist or instrument. Tethering by adhesions (see Diverticular disease, below) may make insertion hazardous or impossible; *force is not the answer.*

'N' or spiral sigmoid looping

Looping of the sigmoid by the endoscope can be anything from a minor upward deviation (sometimes a fixed kink due to adhesions from hysterectomy or previous diverticulitis) to a huge loop reaching toward the diaphragm in some patients with a redundant or megacolon. The exact shape will vary from moment to moment according to the constraints of the abdomen, the mesenteries and the activities of the endoscopist propelling or twisting the colonoscope. Most sigmoid loops are a 3D spiral, the 'N'-type mainly rotating around the left side of the abdomen, whereas the 'alpha'-type rotates initially to the right side.

Removal of the sigmoid loop is essential. Initially this is to help passage into the descending colon. Most of the pain and difficulties experienced subsequently in a colonoscopy—while passing the proximal colon (splenic flexure, transverse colon and hepatic flexure)—also stem from recurrent or persistent N-looping in the sigmoid. Sigmoid looping removes the motive power of the endoscopist's inward push unless the loop can be removed or at least minimized. It is for this reason that, when inserting through the proximal colon, repeated straightening of the sigmoid colon can still be so important.

Straightening out sigmoid N-spiral loops involves pulling back with twist (usually clockwise) to assist in undoing the spiral element. For shorter loops it is worth attempting this during passage through the sigmoid colon, or certainly when the sigmoid–descending junction is reached, so as to attempt direct or 'straight scope' passage to the descending colon, as described above. Although it is worth the endoscopist trying one or two withdrawal movements to shorten the N-loop, especially near the apex of the sigmoid colon but also at any obvious fold or bend which allows 'hooking', often there is little to be done until the sigmoid junction is reached and an attempt can be made at the 'clockwise twist and withdrawal' maneuver, described above. With a longer colon, complete removal of the N-loop may be difficult until the instrument tip has reached well up the descending and nearly to (or around) the splenic flexure, giving adequate purchase for forcible withdrawal. Hand pressure by the assistant in the left lower abdomen often helps by reducing or minimizing the size of the loop (see Fig. 6.36), acting as a buffer to transmit more of the inward push on the shaft toward the descending colon. If the assistant can actually feel the loop, the objective is to reduce it back toward the pelvis (i.e. with downward as well as inward pressure).

The alpha loop and maneuver

A long sigmoid colon may be pushed spontaneously into an 'alpha loop' configuration (Fig. 6.46). From the endoscopist's point of view, an alpha loop is a blessing, since its shape means that there is no acute bend between the sigmoid and descending colon, so the splenic flexure can be reached rapidly and relatively painlessly. If, during insertion, no particularly acute flexure is encountered in the sigmoid colon and the instrument appears to be sliding in a long way without problems or acute angulations, it can be suspected that an alpha loop is being formed. If so (especially if confirmed on fluoroscopy or the 3D imager) it is essential to pass on to the proximal descending colon or splenic flexure at 90 cm (sometimes even around the splenic flexure into the transverse colon) *before* trying any withdrawal/straightening maneuver. Even though the patient has mild stretch pain, push on (Fig. 6.47c) and steer carefully until the tip has passed through

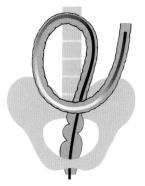

Fig. 6.46 An alpha loop.

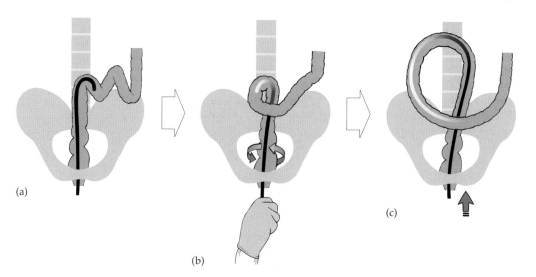

(a)

(b)

(c)

Fig. 6.47 (a) During sigmoid insertion … (b) … if the tip can be made to point to the caecum … (c) … rotate anti-clockwise and push in for the 'alpha' maneuver.

the fluid-filled descending colon to the splenic flexure, reached at 90 cm (Fig. 6.48). Applying normal sigmoid straightening maneuvers half-way round an alpha loop is a potential mistake, since this may cause the alpha configuration to rotate back into an N-spiral loop configuration, with much greater difficulty in reaching up the descending colon.

An alpha loop forms in only 10% of colonoscopies, as shown by our 3D imager studies. Endoscopists who claim 'frequently' to form an alpha loop are shown, when they demonstrate their technique under fluoroscopy or the 3D imager, usually to be 'pushing through' a large N-loop, which they pass with élan—and extra sedation because of the pain involved. A normal short or fixed sigmoid mesocolon (from diverticular disease or any other cause of pericolic adhesions) will not allow formation of an alpha loop.

The alpha maneuver is the intentional formation of an alpha loop. This was a fluoroscopically (or X-ray) monitored routine when using early colonoscopes, and is feasible again with the introduction of 3D magnetic imaging. The principle of the maneuver is to twist the sigmoid colon around into a partial volvulus (see Fig. 6.39). As soon as the instrument is seen to be angling into the distal sigmoid colon towards the caecum (Fig. 6.47a), the shaft is rotated firmly anti-clockwise at every opportunity, so that the angled tip swings and points toward the cecum, pulling the sigmoid colon across with it (Fig. 6.47b). Continued insertion is with as much *anti*-clockwise twist as possible at all stages (avoiding clockwise twist so that the loop does not swing back to the 'N'-position). It is not always possible to achieve the alpha maneuver.

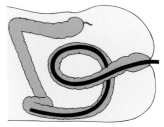

90cm

Fig. 6.48 In an alpha loop the scope runs through the fluid-filled descending colon to the splenic flexure at 90 cm (posterior view).

Straightening an alpha loop

An alpha loop must be removed at some stage, because any loop puts stress and limitation on tip angulation due to friction in the control wires, as well as being uncomfortable for the patient. Most colonoscopists prefer to straighten out the alpha loop as soon as the upper descending colon is safely reached (at 90 cm) and then to pass the splenic flexure with a straightened instrument. However, every colonoscopist has also experienced the chagrin of struggling to reach the descending colon and the frustration of seeing the tip slide back when an attempt is made, too early, to withdraw and straighten the shaft. With current very flexible and fully angling instruments, it is occasionally better to attempt to pass straight on into the proximal transverse colon with the alpha loop in position rather than to straighten it at the splenic flexure and then have difficulty with re-looping.

Alpha loop straightening is by combined withdrawal and strong clockwise de-rotation. Slightly withdrawing the shaft initially reduces the size of the loop and makes de-rotation easier, but

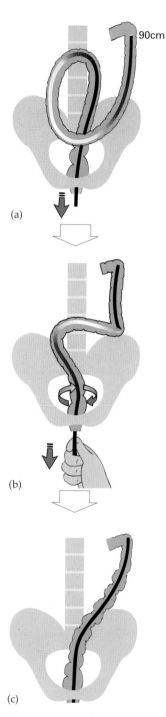

90cm

(a)

(b)

(c)

Fig. 6.49 (a) An alpha loop ... (b)... de-rotates with clockwise twist and withdrawal ... (c)... to straighten completely.

the tip can start to slide down the descending colon. De-rotation alone will undo the alpha volvulus of the sigmoid into the 'N' position, but does not reduce the size of the loop. The two actions must be combined by simultaneously pulling back and twisting the whole instrument (Fig. 6.49). Strong clockwise twist during the alpha straightening process will tend to push the tip inward toward the splenic flexure, so any tendency of the tip to slip back can usually be stopped by applying more twist and less pull. Twisting forces are not harmful to the colonoscope.

De-rotation should be easy and atraumatic. If straightening the loop proves difficult or the patient has more than the slightest discomfort the situation should be reassessed. Adhesions can make de-rotation difficult and occasionally impossible. Do not use force. The sigmoid loop that has formed may not be a true alpha loop but a 'reversed alpha', which can form when there is persistent descending mesocolon and freely mobile left colon (see Fig. 6.41). This reversed loop may need anti-clockwise de-rotation during straightening and, in the absence of imaging, the endoscopist must judge this by *feel* (and results).

Alpha—a 'good' sigmoid loop

- *Insertion is easy, without angulations.*
- *Carry on pushing until 90 cm.*
- *Only then pull back with anti-clockwise twist.*
- *At 50–60 cm the shaft should be straight.*

Atypical sigmoid loops and the 'reversed alpha'

'Atypical' spiral loops can form when colon attachments are unusually mobile, particularly those of the descending colon (see below). Whereas normally the retroperitoneal fixation of the descending colon limits movements of the sigmoid, characteristically in a clockwise spiral, the colonoscope may force a mobile colon into an *anti*-clockwise spiral, or even a complex mix of clockwise and anti-clockwise loops. In practical terms this variation should make little difference to the endoscopist, except in the need to apply the correct de-rotational force when pulling back to straighten the loop. An anti-clockwise 'reversed alpha loop' (see Fig. 6.41) may allow the scope tip to slide up into the descending colon nearly as easily as a conventional alpha loop, with no obvious clue that there is anything odd or unusual. Since around 90% of sigmoid loops spiral clockwise, the unsuspecting endoscopist can waste time and make things worse by trying to de-rotate such an atypical loop with clockwise twist. If the 3D imager is being used, the configuration and its solution are obvious. If, as is more usual, the endoscopist is relying on shaft feel and guesswork it is important to try anti-clockwise twist if the sigmoid appears not to be straightening. Very occasionally looping may be so complex that de-rotational twist has to be first one way, then the other.

Instrument shaft loops external to the patient

Rotating the colonoscope to straighten loops may result in shaft loops external to the patient. Because of the negative effect of any loops on instrument handling, especially on torque steering, it is good practice to de-rotate the control body to transfer this loop to the umbilical (see Fig. 6.33). Several (up to three) loops can be accommodated in the umbilical without harm, but sometimes it may be necessary to unplug the instrument from the light source and unravel the umbilical. The alternative for the dexterous endoscopist, and if the instrument is straight, is to de-rotate the external shaft loop while steering the tip into the lumen so that the colonoscope rotates on its axis within the colon; however, if the shaft is not straight the instrument tends to slip back in the process.

Diverticular disease

In severe diverticular disease there may be a narrowed lumen, pericolic adhesions and problems in choosing the correct direction (Fig. 6.50a). However, once the instrument has been laboriously fiddled through the area, the 'splinting' effect of the abnormally rigid sigmoid may facilitate the rest of the examination. In the presence of diverticular disease the secret is extreme patience, with care in visualization and steering, combined with greater than usual use of withdrawal, rotatory or corkscrewing movements. It helps to realize that a close-up view of a diverticulum means that the tip must be deflected to a right-angle (by withdrawal and angulation or twist) to find the lumen (Fig. 6.50b). Using a thinner and more flexible pediatric colonoscope or gastroscope may make an apparently impassable narrow, fixed or angulated sigmoid colon relatively easy to examine— which sometimes also saves the patient from surgery. Having successfully passed severe or angulated sigmoid diverticular disease (especially if it has taken a short scope to do so), it is the endoscopist's worst nightmare if the proximal colon then proves to be long and mobile.

'Underwater colonoscopy' may help passage in some patients with very hypertrophic musculature and redundant mucosal folds in diverticular disease, in whom it can be very difficult to obtain an adequate view. Water can distend a narrow segment better than air, water having the combined advantages of being non-compressible, remaining in the dependent sigmoid colon (rather than the tendency of air to rise and distend only the

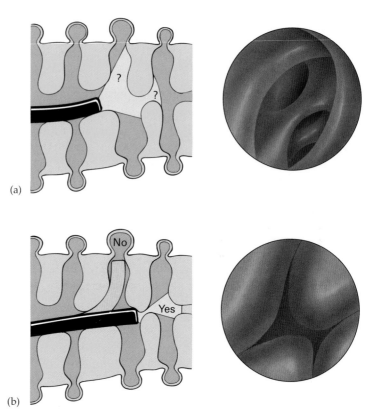

Fig. 6.50 (a) Choosing the correct path can be difficult in diverticular disease … (b)… a circular view is a *diverticulum*—the lumen will be at 90° and is often squashed.

proximal colon in a patient in left lateral position) and also holding the mucosal folds away from the lens to improve the view.

Be prepared to abandon if postoperative or peridiverticular adhesions have fixed the pelvic colon so as to make passage impossible or dangerous. If there is difficulty, if the instrument tip feels fixed and cannot be moved by angling or twisting and the patient complains of pain during attempts at insertion, there is a danger of perforation and the attempt should be abandoned. Sometimes a different endoscope (e.g. pediatric colonoscope or gastroscope) or another endoscopist may succeed. Only a very experienced colonoscopist with very good clinical reasons should put the patient and instrument at risk under these circumstances; usually the most experienced are the most prepared to stop and refer for another form of imaging.

Sigmoid–descending junction

The sigmoid–descending junction is probably the trickiest

point of the examination for most colonoscopists. The sigmoid–descending junction conventionally appears as an acute bend at approximately 40–70 cm. It can be so acute as to appear at first to be a blind ending. In a capacious colon there may be a longitudinal fold pointing toward the correct direction of the lumen, caused by the muscle bulk of a tenia coli (Fig. 6.51); follow the longitudinal fold closely to pass the bend.

At the sigmoid–descending colon junction the tip may reach a fixed (retroperitoneal) point, with the chance of the endoscopist getting control of the mobile sigmoid. As the tip reaches the junction it is worth trying a 'pull-back-and-shortening' move. 'Direct passage' to the descending colon is the ideal, trying to wriggle the tip around the junction without forcing up the sigmoid loop. Experts occasionally, and inexperienced endoscopists frequently, have trouble in achieving this. Typically an overenthusiastic endoscopist, having rounded the sigmoid with panache, will have stretched up a large (iatrogenic) sigmoid spiral N-loop (Fig. 6.52) and created an acute 'hairpin' bend (and extra difficulty) as a result. Being more careful, using less air and frequent withdrawals, should be rewarded by a straighter, even direct, passage from the sigmoid to descending colon (Fig. 6.53).

As soon as the tip is even partially into or around the sigmoid–descending junction try following these steps:

1 *Pull back* the shaft to reduce the loop, which creates a more favorable angle of approach to the junction and also optimizes the instrument mechanics.

2 *Apply abdominal pressure*, the assistant pushing on the left lower abdomen so as to compress the loop or reduce the abdominal space within which it can form.

3 *Deflate the colon* (without losing the view) to shorten it and make it as pliable as possible and help to relax the flaplike inner angle of the sigmoid–descending bend.

4 *'Pre-steer' into the bend*, the tip being steered at the mucosa just before the inner angle (Fig. 6.54), so that on pushing in the pre-

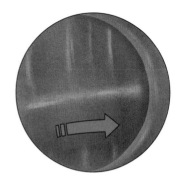

Fig. 6.51 At acute bends a longitudinal bulge (tenia coli) shows the axis to follow.

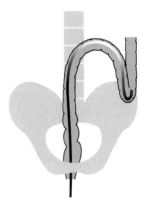

Fig. 6.52 An N-loop stretching up the sigmoid colon.

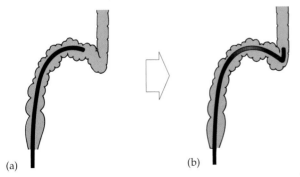

(a)   (b)

Fig. 6.53 (a) Pull back and deflate to keep the sigmoid short … (b)… which may allow direct passage to the descending colon.

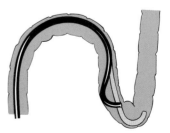

Fig. 6.54 'Pre-steer' before pushing into an acute bend.

steering causes the tip to slip past the angle to point straight at the lumen of the descending colon.

5 *Try shaft twist* in case the configuration allows corkscrewing force to be applied to the tip. Clockwise shaft torque tends to be particularly effective at this point because most sigmoid colons loop in a clockwise spiral—passing anteriorly out of the pelvis, over the pelvic brim and curving laterally and posteriorly into the descending colon (see Fig. 6.35). 'Pull back-with-clockwise twist' is the trick to try. With luck it will simultaneously shorten (pleat/accordion) the sigmoid over the scope shaft and move the tip forward towards the fixed descending colon. When it works the result is a most satisfying feeling for the endoscopist of 'getting something for nothing', quite apart from avoiding pain for the patient.

6 *Changing the patient to the right lateral position* can improve visualization of the sigmoid–descending junction (air rises, water falls) and may sometimes also cause the distal descending colon to drop down into a more favorable configuration for passage. In left lateral position the sigmoid will tend to be crumpled down toward the left flank, with fluid also pooling there. Lying the patient supine may improve the view and (especially in long and mobile sigmoids) the gravitational effect of right lateral position often improves things further still.

7 *Use of force to 'push through' the loop* should once again be the option of last resort. It may be better to warn the patient and push in calculatedly than to struggle on indefinitely or to abandon the procedure when clinical indications for it are strong. Having warned the patient to expect discomfort, a few seconds of careful 'persuasive pressure' may slide the instrument tip successfully around the bend and then allow straightening again. Providing the tip is pointing correctly, it should slip gradually over the mucosa with the 'slide by' appearance of the mucosal vascular pattern traversing the field of view. Continue to push if 'slide by' continues smoothly; stop if the mucosa blanches (indicating excessive local pressure) or if the patient experiences pain (indicating undue strain on the bowel or mesentery). It should not be necessary to push strongly and uncomfortably like this for more than 20–30 seconds at the most; the instrument can then be straightened back rapidly, taking the strain off the colon and its attachments and making the patient comfortable.

In some patients, by good fortune, a spiral 'alpha loop' may have been formed during insertion, which results in easy passage (see pp. 125, 130–1); in other patients with long colons 'push through' reaches up the descending colon anyway, and the endoscopist may be quite unsure as to what has happened. Providing that the patient does not experience pain the exact loop does not matter, so long as the loop (whichever it is) is then removed.

'Clockwise twist and withdrawal' maneuver

A complex simultaneous movement is needed, combining withdrawal, shaft torque and tip steering towards the lumen of the descending colon. After the tip has been successfully hooked around into the descending colon, the colonoscope has to be straightened to allow direct upward passage of the shaft too. Pulling back is effective in doing this because the tip is now retroperitoneal and relatively fixed (Fig. 6.55a). However, an inevitable, but unwanted, consequence of pulling back is that the angulated and 'hooked' tip will impact into the mucosa (Fig. 6.55b). A wrong move at this point can lose the critical retroperitoneal fixation and the instrument will fall back into the sigmoid. Careful interpretation of the close-up view, minimal insufflation, twist, delicate steering movements and patience are all needed to pass in without re-looping (Fig. 6.55c), which results from excessive push or tip impaction. The importance of using clockwise torque rotation to prevent re-looping of the straightened instrument is such that this method of direct passage has been called by Shinya the 'right twist (clockwise) withdrawal' maneuver. The 3D looping of the sigmoid colon into a clockwise spiral is illustrated (Fig. 6.56), showing why shaft torque or twist is so important in making it possible to pass proximally without using force.

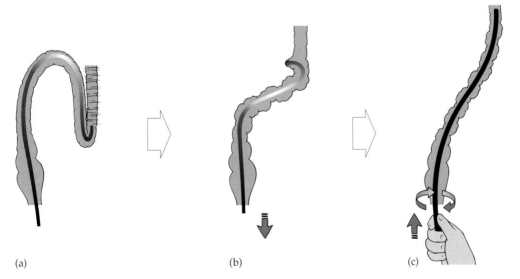

(a)　　　　　　(b)　　　　　　(c)

Fig. 6.55 (a) The tip is hooked into the retroperitoneal descending colon, then pulled back … (b)… and when the endoscope is maximally straightened the tip is redirected … (c)… and the endoscope pushed in, with clockwise twist, into the descending colon.

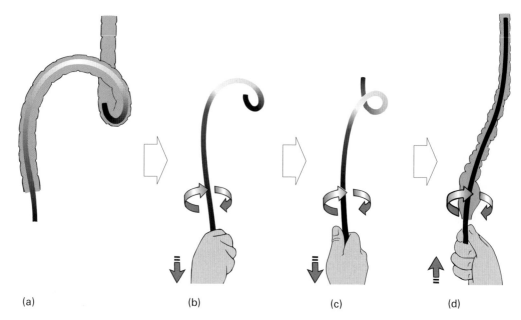

(a)   (b)   (c)   (d)

Fig. 6.56 (a) An N-loop with the tip at the sigmoid–descending colon junction … (b)… twist clockwise and withdraw … (c)… keep twisting and find the lumen of the descending colon … (d)… then push in (still twisting to avoid re-looping).

DESCENDING COLON

The descending colon can be a 20 cm long 'straight', traversed in a few seconds. For the gravitational reasons described above, when the patient is in the left lateral position there is characteristically a horizontal fluid level (Fig. 6.57). Often there is sufficient air interface above the descending colon fluid (or blood in emergency cases) so that the tip can be steered above it. If fluid makes steering difficult, it may be quicker, rather than wasting time suctioning and reinflating, to turn the patient onto the right side to fill the descending colon with air. Apart from this positional trick, and the frequent use of clockwise twist or hand pressure to minimize sigmoid colon re-looping, no particular skills or maneuvers are needed in the average descending colon. Sometimes the descending colon is far from straight and the endoscopist, having struggled through a number of bends and fluid-filled sumps, believes the tip to have reached the proximal colon when the scope has in fact only reached the splenic flexure.

Distal colon mobility and 'reversed' looping

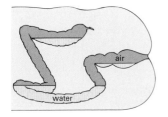

Fig. 6.57 Fluid levels in the left lateral position.

If the descending colon is mobile, without retroperitoneal fixation, the normal anatomy can disappear. At the most extreme, the colonoscope may run through the 'sigmoid' and 'descending' distal colon straight up the midline (see Fig. 6.40), resulting inevitably in a 'reversed splenic flexure' and consequent mechanical problems later in the examination. The endoscopist is alerted to the probability that there is partial fixation, with a descending mesocolon allowing the descending colon to deviate medially, when *anti-clockwise* rotation seems to help insertion at the sigmoid–descending junction. This indicates that an unconventional anti-clockwise spiral loop or 'reversed alpha' has been formed by the instrument (see Fig. 6.41), with the corollary that other oddities may occur during insertion. If possible, the endoscopist tries to use this anti-clockwise twist and the springiness of the colonoscope shaft to push the mobile descending colon outward against the lateral margin of the abdominal cavity. This regains the conventional configuration so that the instrument runs medially (rather than in reverse) around the splenic flexure, and is able to adopt the favorable question-mark shape to reach the cecum. Such apparently mysterious manipulations are understandable to anyone who has done colonoscopy under fluoroscopic control or used the 3D magnetic imager. Straightening can also be achieved, less certainly, by an experienced endoscopist without these aids by the simple expedient of responding to the 'feel' of the endoscope, empirically using whichever twisting movement (in this case anti-clockwise) makes the instrument insert most easily.

SPLENIC FLEXURE

Endoscopic anatomy

The splenic flexure is situated beneath the left costal margin, inaccessible to hand pressure. The colon bends medially and anteriorly around the splenic flexure. The position of the flexure is variably fixed according to the degree of mobility of the fold of peritoneum called the phrenico-colic ligament, which attaches it to the diaphragmatic surface (Fig. 6.58). In some subjects the splenic flexure is tethered up into the left hypochondrium, in others it is relatively free and can be pulled down toward the pelvis (Fig. 6.59). A lax phrenico-colic ligament, a common feature of redundant colons, makes control of the transverse colon difficult by depriving the endoscopist of any fixed point or fulcrum with which to exert leverage during withdrawal maneuvers (the cantilever effect). The configuration of the splenic flexure is also affected by the patient's position, principally because of the effects on it of the transverse colon, which sags down under gravity in the left lateral position or pulls it open in the right lateral position (Fig. 6.60).

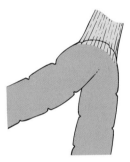

Fig. 6.58 The phrenico-colic ligament.

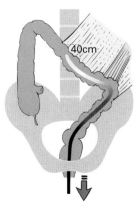

Fig. 6.59 The splenic flexure can pull back to 40 cm if there is a free phrenico-colic ligament.

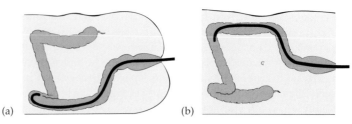

(a)   (b)

Fig. 6.60 (a) In the left lateral position the transverse colon flops down making the splenic flexure acute … (b)… whereas in the right lateral position gravity rounds off the splenic flexure, making it easy to pass.

Insertion around the splenic flexure

The splenic flexure represents the 'half-time' point during colonoscopy and is an excellent moment at which to ensure that the instrument is properly straightened to 50 cm from the anus and under control before tackling the proximal colon. The commonest reason for experiencing problems in the proximal colon is because the colonoscope has been inadequately straightened at the splenic flexure; persistence of loops makes the rest of the procedure progressively more difficult or impossible. If the splenic flexure is passed with straight shaft configuration at 50 cm, using the above rules, the rest of a total colonoscopy insertion should usually be finished within a minute or two. Anyone who frequently finds the proximal colon or hepatic flexure difficult to traverse should apply the '50 cm rule' at the splenic flexure, and is likely to find most of the problem solved once the distal colon has been properly straightened.

Passage around the apex of the splenic flexure is usually obvious because the instrument emerges from fluid into the air-filled, often triangular, transverse colon (Fig. 6.61). However, while the flexible and angled tip section of the colonoscope passes around without effort, the stiffer segment at 10–15 cm at the leading part of the shaft does not follow so easily. This problem is accentuated in the left lateral position, because drooping of the transverse colon causes the splenic flexure to be acutely angled (see Fig. 6.60a) compared with its configuration when opened out by gravity in the right lateral position (see Fig. 6.60b).

To pass the splenic flexure without force or re-looping:

1 *Straighten the scope.* Pull back with the tip hooked around the flexure until the instrument is 40–60 cm from the anus, which both straightens any sigmoid loop and pulls down and rounds-off the flexure. Note that splenic avulsions or capsular tears have been reported, so be *gentle*.

2 *Avoid overangulation of the tip.* Full angulation results in the bending section impacting in the splenic flexure, preventing further insertion (the 'walking-stick handle' effect). Having obtained a view of the transverse colon and pulled back, con-

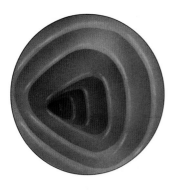

Fig. 6.61 The transverse colon is usually triangular.

sciously de-angulate a little so that the instrument runs around the outside of the bend (see Fig. 6.23), even if this means worsening the view somewhat.

3 *Deflate the colon* slightly to shorten the flexure and make it malleable.

4 *Apply assistant hand pressure* over the sigmoid colon. Any resistance encountered at the splenic flexure is likely to result in stretching upwards of the sigmoid colon into an 'N'-loop or spiral loop, which dissipates more and more of the inward force applied to the shaft as the loop increases (Fig. 6.62). It is immediately obvious to the single-handed endoscopist that such a loop is forming, because the 'one-to-one' relationship between insertion and tip progress is lost—in other words, the shaft is being pushed in but the tip moves little or not at all. Pull back again to restraighten the shaft if this occurs.

5 *Use clockwise torque on the shaft.* As explained above, the clockwise spiral course of the sigmoid colon from the pelvis to its point of fixation in the descending colon means that applying clockwise torque to the colonoscope shaft tends to counteract any looping tendency in the sigmoid colon while pushing in (Fig. 6.63). Clockwise torque will only be effective to keep the shaft straight if any significant looping has been removed and if the descending colon is normally fixed. Because the tip is angulated, applying clockwise shaft torque may affect the luminal view into the transverse colon, and readjustment of the angulation controls may be needed to redirect the tip.

6 *Finally, push in, but slowly.* The instrument tip cannot advance around the splenic flexure without some degree of inward push. So, as well as clockwise twist, continued gentle inward pressure is needed (aggressive pushing simply re-forms the sigmoid loop). All that is needed for success is firm inward pressure on the shaft—which causes gradual millimeter-by-millimeter inward slippage of the tip into the transverse colon. While pushing in it may be possible to deflate again, or it may be necessary to make compensatory movements of the steering controls. A combination of these various maneuvers, together or in sequence, using the angulation controls to 'squirm' the bending section, or the suction valve to aspirate a little more, may help the tip and the stiffer shaft behind it to slide around the splenic flexure.

7 *If it does not work, pull back and start again.* If the tip is not progressing but, from the amount of shaft being inserted, it is obvious that a sigmoid loop is re-forming, pull back and run through all the above actions again before pushing in once more. It may take two or three attempts to achieve success.

8 *If a variable scope is being used,* stiffening it—once the splenic flexure is reached and the instrument is straightened—may stop shaft re-looping in the sigmoid, and let inward push slide the tip straight around into the transverse with remarkable ease.

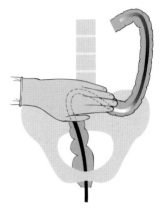

Fig. 6.62 Control sigmoid looping by hand pressure to help pass the splenic flexure.

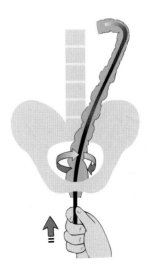

Fig. 6.63 Twist the shaft clockwise while advancing to keep the sigmoid straight.

Summary: passing the splenic flexure

1 *Pull back to straighten the scope.*
2 *Avoid overangulation of the tip.*
3 *Deflate the colon.*
4 *Apply assistant hand pressure.*
5 *Use clockwise torque on the shaft.*
6 *Push in, but slowly.*
7 *Stiffen a variable scope.*
8 *Change position to back or right side—and try again!*

Position change

Patient position change is the most effective secondary trick if the splenic flexure is proving hard to pass. As pointed out earlier, the left lateral position used by most endoscopists has the undesirable effect of causing the transverse colon to flop down (see Fig. 6.60a) and make the splenic flexure acutely angled. Turning the patient to the right lateral position has the opposite effect, the transverse colon sagging to the right side and, together with gravity, pulling the splenic flexure into a smooth curve without any apparent 'flexure' at all (see Fig. 6.60b). Even getting the patient to turn supine has a significant gravitational effect and, since this is an easier move to make, it is worth trying the patient on their back before a full right lateral change.

Change of position does take a few seconds to achieve, and the patient has to be returned to the left lateral position to inflate and visualize the proximal colon properly and to reach the cecum. It is also cumbersome if the patient is obese, disabled or oversedated. We therefore change position if 'stuck' at the splenic flexure for over 60 seconds or so, allowing several attempts at direct passage, first in the left lateral position, then the supine, before full rotation to the right. The ability to perform postural changes easily is an additional reason for reducing routine sedation (or avoiding it altogether when possible).

Position change can be made into a simple routine.
1 *Change hands, to hold the instrument control body in the right hand.*
2 *The endoscopist's left hand raises the patient's lower foot, which lifts both legs.*
3 *The shaft is slid through to the other side of the legs.*
4 *The patient can then turn over.*
Providing the shaft is kept away from the patient's heels there is nothing to go wrong. The whole position change maneuver takes at most 20–30 seconds in a lightly sedated patient.

The split stiffening or 'overtube'

A stiffening overtube, sometimes called a 'splinting device', may hold a looping sigmoid colon straight and allow easier passage into the proximal colon. As well as its use for stiffening a looping sigmoid colon, an overtube can be invaluable for exchanging colonoscopes or removing multiple polypectomy specimens. The overtube can only be inserted when the sigmoid colon has been completely straightened and the tip of the instrument is in the proximal descending colon or splenic flexure. Use of overtubes has largely fallen out of fashion because of their cumbersome nature and unpredictability. With the use of 3D imaging, allowing uncontrollable sigmoid looping to be accurately assessed and straightened, it is possible that overtubes will once again be found to be an occasionally useful accessory.

The original extremely stiff (wire-reinforced) overtubes had disadvantages that discouraged most endoscopists from using them. The tube had to be on the instrument before starting (or the endoscope completely withdrawn before putting it on), and insertion was sometimes traumatic, with perforations reported. A soft-plastic split overtube overcomes all of these disadvantages, and prototype atraumatic versions made of frictionless and very flexible plastic material (Gortex) have proved effective. The split overtube is placed over the shaft of the colonoscope after this has been straightened to 50 cm at the splenic flexure (Fig. 6.64a). The overtube split is sealed with adhesive tape and lubricated with jelly (Fig. 6.64b), then inserted (without fluoroscopy) as far into or through the shortened sigmoid colon as proves easy and comfortable for the patient (Fig. 6.64c).

Resistance to insertion of an overtube means risky impaction against a fold, loop or flexure; discomfort means the same. Both are indications that further insertion or use of force could be dangerous. The handle of the overtube is held by the assistant and the shaft of the colonoscope pushed in through it (Fig. 6.65). As soon as the colonoscope has been passed in satisfactorily (or at once if the overtube cannot be inserted successfully) it takes only a few seconds to remove the split overtube again, strip off the tape and return to normal handling of the instrument.

The 'reversed' splenic flexure

Atypical passage around the splenic flexure occurs in about 1 patient in 20, if imaging is available to see what is happening. The instrument tip passes *laterally* rather than medially around the splenic flexure, because the descending colon has moved centrally on a mesocolon (Fig. 6.66) (see p. 109). This is of more than academic interest because, having passed laterally round the flexure and displaced the descending colon medially, the advancing instrument forces the transverse colon down into a deep loop. The instrument is then mechanically under stress and difficult to steer, and the hepatic flexure is approached from below at a disadvantageous angle, making it difficult to reach the

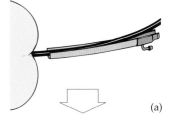

(a)

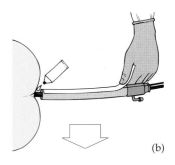

(b)

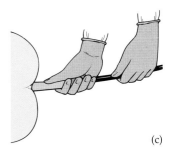

(c)

Fig. 6.64 (a) Insert the split overtube onto the colonoscope shaft ... (b)... seal the slit with sticky tape and lubricate ... (c)... and slide the overtube in; keep the endoscope stationary with the other hand.

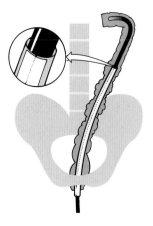

Fig. 6.65 A split overtube inserted to 30–40 cm prevents looping of the sigmoid.

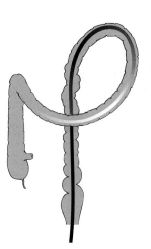

Fig. 6.66 A 'reversed' splenic flexure will result in a deep transverse loop.

cecum and virtually impossible to steer into the ileo-cecal valve. With a reversed splenic loop, even when the instrument tip can be hooked onto the hepatic flexure, the sheer bulkiness of the reversed loop configuration actively holds down the transverse loop, stopping it being straightened and lifted up into the ideal 'question-mark' shape.

De-rotation of a reversed splenic flexure loop may be possible and will avoid these problems later in the examination. This can be done by twisting the shaft strongly anti-clockwise (rather than the usual clockwise twist), usually after withdrawing the tip to the splenic flexure. The subsequent examination is so much quicker, and also more comfortable for the patient, making the time spent worthwhile. Anti-clockwise de-rotation makes the tip pivot around the phrenico-colic suspensory ligament and swing medially (Fig. 6.67a). After that, by maintaining anti-clockwise torque while pushing in, the instrument can be made to pass across the transverse colon in the usual configuration, forcing the descending colon back laterally against the abdominal wall (Fig. 6.67b).

This anti-clockwise straightening maneuver is most easily performed under imaging but is also quite feasible by feel, using these guidelines and a little imagination whenever possible atypical looping is suspected in the proximal colon. A reversed splenic flexure/mobile descending colon is the most frequent reason for an unexpectedly difficult adult or pediatric colonoscopy. It hap-

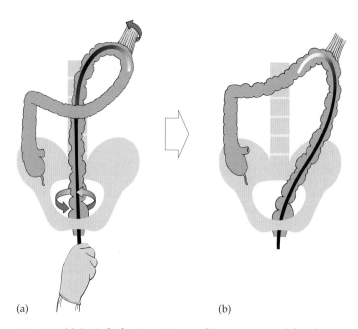

(a) (b)

Fig. 6.67 (a) Anti-clockwise rotation … (b)… swings a mobile colon back to a normal position.

pens more commonly in children due to the relative elasticity of the attachments of the colon in childhood. Sometimes the best solution, if the problem is suspected but imaging is not available and attempts at anti-clockwise de-rotation have failed, is simply to get a move on and to 'push through' more vigorously than usual (if necessary with extra sedation) and then to abandon the procedure as soon as a reasonable view of the right colon has been obtained. For the reasons given above, if a reversed splenic loop is present, it is rare to be able to enter the ileum without successful de-rotation and straightening, because the looped and stressed instrument will not angulate sufficiently. If ileoscopy is essential and a reversed loop is present it is likely to be necessary to pull the instrument out to 50 cm at the splenic flexure, attempt anti-clockwise de-rotation and pass in again; failing to do this and simply trying to angulate the tip forcibly is likely to stress the bending section, and not succeed.

TRANSVERSE COLON

Endoscopic anatomy

In 30% of subjects the transverse colon lies anteriorly just beneath the abdominal wall, held forward by the vertebral bodies, the duodenum and pancreas, and relates to the left and right lobes of the liver (Fig. 6.68). It is enveloped in a double fold of peritoneum called the transverse mesocolon (Fig. 6.69), which originates from the posterior wall of the abdomen and hangs down posterior to the stomach, varying considerably in length. In a barium enema study, the transverse colon of 62% of females drooped down into the pelvis, compared to only 26% of males. This longer transverse loop largely accounts for the 10–20 cm greater mean colon length found in women despite their smaller stature (total colon length was 80–180 cm) and probably also contributes to our experience that 70% of difficult colonoscopies are in females (previous hysterectomy making only a small contribution). The depth of the looped transverse colon also affects the angle at which the endoscope approaches the hepatic flexure, in the same way that the size of the sigmoid colon loop causes an acute sigmoid–descending colon bend. Because the transverse mesocolon (Fig. 6.70a) is broad-based it does not usually allow a gamma loop to form (Fig. 6.70b). From an anatomical and endoscopic viewpoint, the hepatic flexure is a nearly 180° hairpin bend, similar in many respects to the bend at the sigmoid–descending junction but more constant in its fixation and more voluminous.

The triangular configuration of the transverse colon (see Fig. 6.61) depends on the relative thinness of the circular muscles compared with the longitudinal muscle bundles of the teniae coli (Fig. 6.71). In some patients (such as those with longstanding colitis but also some normals) the circular musculature is thicker

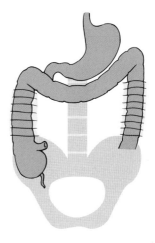

Fig. 6.68 The transverse colon is anterior, over the duodenum and pancreas; the descending and ascending colon are fixed retroperitoneally.

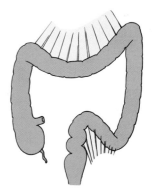

Fig. 6.69 Colon mesenteries—the transverse and sigmoid mesocolons.

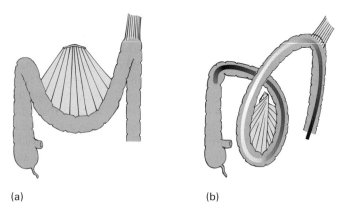

Fig. 6.70 (a) Transverse mesocolon. (b) A gamma loop.

and the transverse colon can be tubular. Both at the mid-transverse flexure and at the hepatic flexure a true 'face-on' view of the haustral folds may be obtained; these present a characteristic 'knife-edge' or 'ladder' appearance (Fig. 6.72); it is therefore easy to confuse the mid-transverse flexure with the hepatic flexure. The mid-transverse bend should be less voluminous, show no blue/gray liver patch and may show transmitted cardiac (double) or aortic (single) pulsation; it can also be distinguished by imaging, local palpation of the anterior abdominal wall or transillumination (if the room is darkened).

Insertion through the transverse colon

Insertion around the transverse should be easy, *unless* the sigmoid colon has also looped, so reducing inward transmitted pressure on the shaft. However, in the mid-transverse colon the angled scope tip often forms a surprisingly sharp bend, pushing the loop downward into the pelvis. A drooping transverse colon, frequently found in females and those with long colons, inevitably results in greater friction resistance to passage; the force required then results in sigmoid looping as well. This combination can be a major obstacle to 'push and go' endoscopists who have not learned the wisdom of shortening and controlling colon loops.

The antimesenteric tenia coli may in-fold into the colon in a voluminous transverse colon, acting as a useful pointer to the correct longitudinal axis to follow—rather like the white line down the centre of a road (Fig. 6.73). Appreciating this is particularly helpful at very acute angulations, where a tenia coli can be followed blindly to push round the bend and see the lumen beyond (Fig. 6.74).

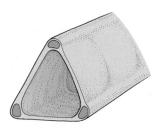

Fig. 6.71 The triangular configuration is due to the teniae coli.

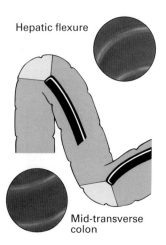

Fig. 6.72 Similar 'knife-like' haustra are seen at the mid-transverse colon and hepatic flexure.

After passing the mid-point of the transverse, it may be slow and difficult to 'climb the hill' up the proximal limb of the looped transverse colon (Fig. 6.75a). The most important maneuver is to *pull back* repeatedly. The tip, being hooked around the transverse loop, lifts up and flattens the transverse (Fig. 6.75b) so that the tip often advances as the shaft is withdrawn—the phenomenon of 'paradoxical movement'. Substantial and repeated in-and-out movements (like playing a trombone) may be needed, the instrument advancing little by little towards the hepatic flexure. Hand pressure can be helpful, whether over the sigmoid colon during inward push or in the left hypochondrium to lift up the transverse loop. Deflation of the colon, torquing movements and even change of position (usually to the left lateral position, sometimes to the supine, right lateral or even prone positions) can all also help. When the tip is established in the proximal transverse colon anti-clockwise torque often helps it to advance toward the hepatic flexure; this useful phenomenon results from flattening out of the *anti-clockwise* spiral formed by the shaft running anteriorly and medially around the splenic flexure from the descending colon to the transverse colon.

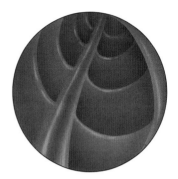

Fig. 6.73 The longitudinal bulge of a tenia coli shows the axis of the colon.

To reach the hepatic flexure

1 *Pull back to lift up the transverse loop.*
2 *Deflate.*
3 *Try anti-clockwise twist.*
4 *Try hand pressure in the left hypochondrium …*
5 *… or hand pressure over the sigmoid.*

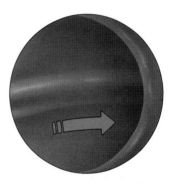

Fig. 6.74 Follow the longitudinal bulge (tenia coli) round an acute bend.

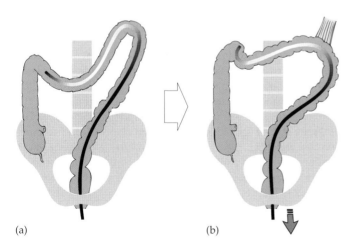

(a)   (b)

Fig. 6.75 (a) If passage up the proximal transverse is difficult …
(b)… pull back to lift and shorten.

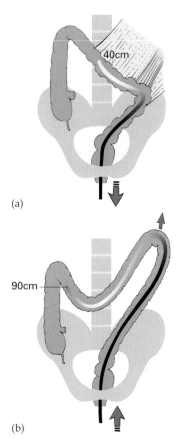

(a)

(b)

Fig. 6.76 (a) If the phrenico-colic ligament is lax, withdrawal maneuvers are ineffective … (b)… and pushing in simply re-forms the loop.

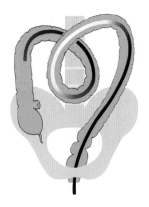

Fig. 6.77 A gamma loop in a redundant transverse colon.

A mobile splenic flexure may adversely affect 'transverse lift' maneuvers. The fulcrum or cantilever effect caused by the phrenico-colic ligament fixing the normal splenic flexure is crucial. In some patients this attachment is lax, allowing the splenic flexure to be pulled back to 40 cm (rather than the usual 50 cm) (Fig. 6.76a); the colon is then found to be hypermobile and unresponsive to any of the normally effective withdrawal or twisting movements (Fig. 6.76b). When this occurs the use of force is ineffectual, but deflation, hand pressure, posturing (usually to the right lateral position) and gentle perseverance will eventually coax the tip up to the hepatic flexure. Simple aggression and force usually worsen things irrevocably, whereas subtlety and patience (eventually) win.

A 'gamma loop' may form in a very long redundant transverse colon (Fig. 6.77), as can be well seen using the 3D imager. A gamma loop is large and rarely removable, both because of its sheer size (conflicting with the small intestine and other organs during attempted de-rotation) and because colon mobility makes it difficult to find any point where angulation will anchor the tip. The instrument therefore falls back each time it is withdrawn. On the rare occasions that a gamma loop is successfully removed, this is by combined withdrawal and very strong twist (clockwise or counterclockwise) to lift up the transverse colon into a more conventional position. Having the 3D imager available greatly increases the chance of success, because it shows very obviously which direction twist to apply, and whether the maneuver is starting to work. It is usually impossible to enter the ileo-cecal valve with a gamma loop in position, because friction stops the instrument tip angulating sufficiently.

Hand pressure over the transverse or sigmoid colon

Hand pressure is helpful in about 30% of transverse colons, reducing the tendency for scope looping within the abdominal cavity and encouraging as straight a line as possible to the cecum. The rationale for pressure in the lower left abdomen over the looping sigmoid colon has been described (see Fig. 6.62). The tendency of the sigmoid to re-loop at all stages of the examination has also been mentioned. Because of this tendency, hand pressure over the sigmoid colon is a good bet whenever the instrument is looping, and its application has therefore been called *'non-specific'* hand pressure.

Brief and gentle initial hand pressure may affect the transverse colon if it reaches near enough to the abdominal wall to be accessible. This maneuver has been called *'specific'* hand pressure. In the proximal colon, at any time that a few extra centimeters of insertion are needed, but cannot be achieved, try abdominal hand pressure—first 'non-specific' (in the left lower abdomen) but, if this fails, 'specifically' according to the results of local palpation.

First, the transverse loop should be pulled up, then aspiration collapses the colon and brings the flexure nearer still. It is at this point that the final action to reach up to or around the flexure may be 'specific' assistant hand pressure—empirically applied to one of the following :

• left hypochondrium region (to push the whole loop toward the hepatic flexure);
• mid-abdomen (to counteract the sagging transverse colon (Fig. 6.78);
• right hypochondrium (to impact directly on the hepatic flexure).

HEPATIC FLEXURE

Passing the hepatic flexure is helped by a sequence of actions:

1 *Assess from a distance* the correct direction around the flexure because, after the tip reaches into it, it will be so close to the opposing mucosa that it is very difficult to steer except by a predetermined plan. At all costs avoid impacting the tip forcibly against the opposing wall or it will catch in the haustral folds and there will be no view at all.

2 *Ask the patient to breathe in* (and hold the breath), which lowers the diaphragm, and often the flexure too.

3 *Aspirate air carefully* from the hepatic flexure, to collapse it toward, but not actually onto, the tip as it moves around (Fig. 6.79).

4 *Steer the tip blindly* in the previously determined direction around the arc of the flexure. Since the hepatic flexure is very acute, it takes some confidence to angulate nearly 180° around in the same direction without seeing well (Fig. 6.80). Use both angulation controls simultaneously to achieve full angulation; adding clockwise twist may be helpful.

5 *Withdraw the instrument* substantially for up to 30–50 cm to lift up the transverse colon and straighten out the colonoscope (Fig. 6.81a,b) for passage into the ascending colon.

6 *Aspirate air again* once the ascending colon is seen, in order to shorten the colon and drop the colonoscope down toward the cecum (Fig. 6.81c).

Summary: passing the hepatic flexure

1 Assess *the correct direction.*
2 *Ask the patient to breathe in.*
3 *Aspirate air to collapse the flexure.*
4 *Angulate the tip 180° around (often blindly).*
5 *Withdraw the instrument substantially.*
6 *Aspirate again to drop the scope down to the cecum.*

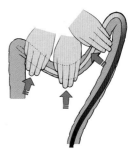

Fig. 6.78 'Specific' hand pressure may elevate the transverse colon.

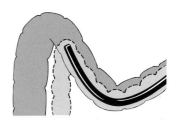

Fig. 6.79 Aspirate to shrink the hepatic flexure towards the scope.

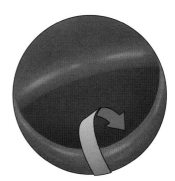

Fig. 6.80 Suction toward, then angle acutely (180°) around the acute hepatic flexure.

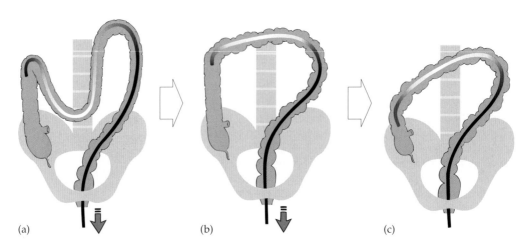

(a)   (b)   (c)

Fig. 6.81 (a) When around the hepatic flexure and viewing the ascending colon … (b)… pull back to straighten … (c)… and aspirate to collapse the colon and pass toward the cecum.

A combination of these maneuvers is used simultaneously. Aspiration brings the hepatic flexure toward the tip until the inner fold of the flexure can be passed, the colonoscope is withdrawn (either by manipulation of the shaft or by the endoscopist pulling the colonoscope out, using both hands simultaneously to work the angulation controls) and the tip is steered maximally around until it can be sucked down into the ascending colon. A parallel has already been drawn between the 'hook, withdraw and clockwise twist' situation in the transverse loop and hepatic flexure and the 'right twist and withdrawal' method of shortening the sigmoid N-loop at the sigmoid–descending colon angle; the same instrument maneuvers apply to both, except that they must be exaggerated at the hepatic flexure because of its larger dimensions.

Position change is another trick that helps coax the colonoscope tip into and around the hepatic flexure. Change the patient's position (to supine, prone or sometimes even right lateral positions) if the usual left lateral position has been ineffective. Using brute force rarely pays off, since the combined sigmoid and transverse colon loops can take up most of the length of the colonoscope shaft. With the instrument really straightened at the hepatic flexure, only about 70 cm of the shaft should remain in the patient; this is one of the situations where a distance check helps to ensure a straight colonoscope and results in easy and painless insertion.

Is it the hepatic flexure—or may it be the splenic? A final, embarrassing, point is that if things are not working out at the hepatic flexure after applying the various tips, the colonoscope may actually still be at the splenic flexure. In a redundant colon it is possible to be overoptimistic and get hopelessly lost. The clue to this is often that the hepatic flexure (in left lateral position) is dry or air-filled, whereas the splenic is likely to be fluid-filled.

ASCENDING COLON AND ILEO-CECAL REGION

Endoscopic anatomy

The ascending colon is posteriorly placed at its origin from the hepatic flexure, but then runs anteriorly so that where it joins the cecum it is just under the anterior abdominal wall and usually accessible to finger palpation or transillumination. In 90% of subjects, the ascending colon and cecum are predictably fixed retroperitoneally, but the remainder may be mobile on a persistent mesocolon, with correspondingly variable positions.

At the pole of the cecum the three teniae coli may fuse around the appendix (crow's-foot or 'Mercedes Benz' sign) (Fig. 6.82), but the anatomy is somewhat variable. Between the teniae coli and the marked cecal haustra there can be cavernous out-pouchings, which are difficult to examine. The appendix orifice is normally an unimpressive slit, which is often crescentic because the appendix is folded around the cecum. The appendix is characteristically flexed around toward the center of the abdomen, thereby giving guidance as to the likely site of entry of the ileum (see 'Finding the ileo-cecal valve', below). Only rarely is the appendix orifice seen straight-on as a tube, probably when the cecum is fully mobile. The appendix may sometimes be less than obvious in a local whirl of mucosal folds. The operated appendix usually looks no different unless it has been invaginated into a stump, when it can sometimes resemble a polyp (take care—perhaps take a biopsy but do not attempt polypectomy!).

The ileo-cecal valve is on the prominent ileo-cecal fold encircling the cecum about 5 cm back from its pole. Unfortunately for the endoscopist, the orifice of the valve is often a slit on the invisible upstream or 'cecal' aspect of the ileo-cecal fold. The most the endoscopist normally sees is the slight bulge of the upper lip. It is therefore rare to see the orifice directly without specific close-up maneuvers.

Reaching the cecum

On seeing the ascending colon the temptation is to push in, but this usually results in the transverse loop re-forming and the tip sliding back. The secret is to *deflate*; the resulting collapse of the capacious hepatic flexure and ascending colon will drop the tip downward toward the cecum (see Fig. 6.81c); it also lowers the position of the hepatic flexure relative to the splenic flexure and with this mechanical advantage, pushing inward should

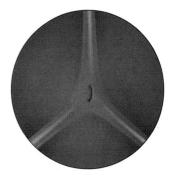

Fig. 6.82 Appendix orifice.

become effective. Aspirate, and steer carefully down the center of the deflating lumen, then push the last few centimeters into the cecum. If it proves difficult to reach the last few centimeters to the cecal pole, change the patient's position to prone (even a partial position change of 20–30° may help) or, if that does not work, change to supine position. Once in the cecum, the bowel can be reinflated to get a view.

The cecum can be voluminous with pronounced haustral in-fold-ings and tendency to spasm making it confusing to examine. In particular, it is possible to be mistaken about whether the pole has actually been reached. One catch is that the ileo-cecal valve fold, the major circumferential fold at the junction of the ascend-ing colon and the cecum—on which is situated the giveaway bulge of the valve—has a tendency to be in tonic spasm. The contracted fold may easily be mistaken by the unwary either for the appendix orifice or for the ileo-cecal valve. Insufflating and pushing in with the instrument tip and/or using extra intra-venous antispasmodic medication will reveal the cavernous cecal pole beyond.

Be careful to identify landmarks before assuming 'total colonoscopy' has been performed. The appendix orifice or ileo-cecal valve should be identified as landmarks, with or without imaging; also use right iliac fossa transillumination (Fig. 6.83) or finger palpation indenting the cecal region (Fig. 6.84) to confirm location of the tip. At the same time the colonoscope should, after withdrawal, be at 70–80 cm. The cecal pole is often difficult to examine, is not always completely clean and is sometimes in tonic spasm; a 'too good to be true' appearance may therefore actually be only the ascending colon or even the hepatic flexure. Inability to locate the ileo-cecal valve opening and noting that the shaft distance on withdrawal is only at 60–70 cm should warn of this possibility.

Finding the ileo-cecal valve

The 'appendix trick' or 'bow and arrow' sign is an ingenious way of finding the ileo-cecal valve—and simultaneously entering it too—a 'double whammy' when it works first time, as it often does!

1 Find the appendix orifice.

2 Imagine an arrow pointing in the direction of the appendix lumen (Fig. 6.85a)

3 Angulate in that direction and pull back (still angled) for about 3–4 cm.

4 At this point expect the proximal lip of the ileo-cecal valve to start to ride up over the lens, with shiny bumps of close-up ileal villi apparent, rather than the mirror-smooth crypt-spotted colon mucosa. (Fig. 6.85b).

5 Slow completely, insufflate and twist or angle gently to wangle into the ileum.

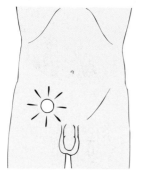

Fig. 6.83 Transillumination deep in the iliac fossa suggests the cecum.

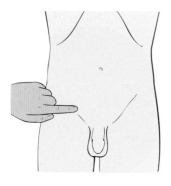

Fig. 6.84 Finger pressure in the right iliac fossa indents the cecum.

The 'appendix trick' works only when (as it usually is) the appendix angulates in the direction of the center of the abdomen—from which direction the ileum also enters the cecum. The appendix effectively acts as an indicator of direction (rather as an airport windsock does for a pilot to indicate wind direction). After appendicectomy or when the cecum is mobile and the appendix can be 'straight-on', there is no indication.

The alternative way of finding the valve is to pull back about 8–10 cm from the cecal pole and then to look for the first prominent circular haustral fold, around 5 cm back from the pole. Somewhere on this 'ileo-cecal' fold will be the tell-tale thickening or bulge of the valve. A common mistake is to look for the valve when the endoscope tip is in the cecal pole, rather than pulling back to the mid-ascending colon to get a proper overall view from a distance. Looking at this ileo-cecal fold, with the cecum moderately inflated, one part of it should be seen to be less perfectly concave than the rest. It may be simply flattened out, bulge in (especially on deflation, when it often bulges more obviously and may bubble or issue ileal contents), show a characteristic 'buttock-like' double bulge or, less commonly, have obvious protuberant lips or a 'volcano' appearance (Fig. 6.86). It is rather uncommon to see the actual slit orifice or pouting lips of the valve straight on, because the opening is normally on the cecal side of the ileo-cecal fold. The best the endoscopist can usually achieve is a partial, close-up and tangential view, and only often after careful maneuvering. Change of patient position may be helpful if the initial view is poor or disadvantageous for tip entry.

Entering the ileum

'Direct entry' into the ileum is made easier by a combination of actions:

1 *Rehearse at a distance* (about 10 cm back from the cecal pole) the easiest movements, preferably combining shaft twist and down-angulation to point the tip toward the valve (Fig. 6.87a). If possible rotate the endoscope so that the valve lies in the downward (6-o'clock) position relative to the tip, because this allows entry with an easy downward angulation movement (lateral or oblique movements are awkward single-handedly) and because the tip air outlet is situated below the lens, but needs to enter the valve first in order to open up the ileum on insufflation.

2 *Pass the colonoscope tip* in over the ileo-cecal valve fold in the region of the valvular bulge and angle in toward the valve (Fig. 6.87b). Overshoot a little, so that the action of angulation directs the tip into the opening, not short of it.

3 *Deflate the cecum* partially to make the valve supple (Fig. 6.87b).

4 *Pull back the scope*, angling downward until the tip catches in the soft lips of the valve, resulting in a 'red-out' of transil-

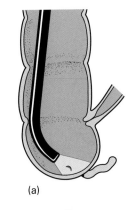

(a)

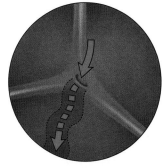

(b)

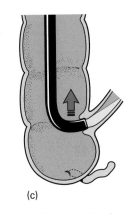

(c)

Fig. 6.85 (a) Angle in the direction of the appendix lumen … (b)… and pull back until the proximal lip of the ileo-cecal valve rides up into view.

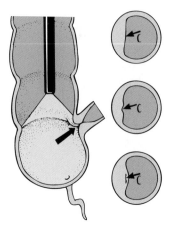

Fig. 6.86 The ileo-cecal valve is a bulge on the ileo-cecal fold and can be a single bulge, double bulge or 'volcano'.

luminated tissue (Fig. 6.87c), typically with the tell-tale granular appearance of the villous surface in close-up (as opposed to the pale shine of colonic mucosa).

5 *On seeing the 'red-out', freeze all movement*, then

6 *Insufflate air* to open the lips (Fig. 6.87d) and wait—gently twisting or angling the scope a few millimeters if necessary until the direction of the ileal lumen becomes apparent; if considerable angulation has been used to enter the valve *de*-angulation may be needed to straighten things out and let the tip slide in.

7 *Multiple attempts may be needed for success*—both in locating the valve and entering the ileum, if necessary rotating to slightly different parts of the ileo-cecal fold, hooking over it and pulling back to pass the area repeatedly. On each successive attempt try to learn from the problems of the previous one, fining down tip movements to a centimeter or two and a few degrees either way. Change of position may also help.

The biopsy forceps can be used as a guide wire. If only a distant, partial or uncertain view can be obtained of the ileal bulge or opening, it is usually possible to use the biopsy forceps to locate and then pass into the opening of the valve (Fig. 6.88), either to obtain a blind biopsy or to act as an 'anchor'. The forceps fix the position of the tip relative to the valve and facilitate endoscope passage through it on the guide-wire principle. Even if entry into the ileum is not intended, the opened forceps can be used to hook back the bulge of the upper lip of the valve to visualize the ileal opening and make identification certain; suggestive bulges or flattened areas can be identified misleadingly on more distal folds.

Entry into the ileum can be in retroflexion. This 'last ditch' maneuver is only likely to work in a huge colon and if the scope is completely straightened and responsive. It is a useful option when the ileo-cecal valve is slit-like and invisible from above (Fig. 6.89). Retrovert the tip to visualize and then to enter the valve from

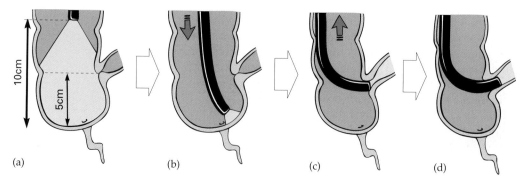

(a)   (b)   (c)   (d)

Fig. 6.87 (a) Locate the ileo-cecal valve (preferably at 6 o'clock) … (b)… pass in and angulate and deflate slightly … (c)… pull back until the 'red-out' is seen … (d)… and insufflate to open the valve.

below (Fig. 6.90a). Very acute angulation of the colonoscope tip is needed, with maximum up/down and lateral angulation, and often some twist of the shaft as well. Fairly forceful inward push may be needed to impact low enough in the cecal pole to visualize the valve. When using video-endoscopes the extra length of the bending section due to the CCD means that the tip retroverts into mid-ascending colon. In those few cases that the valve can be seen, pull back to impact the tip within it (Fig. 6.90b), insufflate to open the lips and de-angulate and pull back further to enter the ileum, with or without use of the forceps (Fig. 6.90c).

Problems in finding or entering the ileo-cecal valve occur for a number of reasons. The endoscope may be in the hepatic flexure, not the cecum. Even if the tip is in the right place, the chosen 'bulge' on the ileo-cecal valve may not be correct; some valve openings are entirely flat and slit-like, effectively invisible on the reverse side of the fold. Aiming the lens at the center of the endoscope tip exactly at the slit may mean that the rest of the tip impacts against the upper lip and cannot pass in (Fig. 6.91), which is why overshooting the opening slightly will let the angled tip edge in successfully even though the initial view is less good.

Those cases of active inflammatory disease (especially Crohn's) where the colonoscopist wants to see the terminal ileum are those where the valve is most likely to be narrowed and, although a limited view may be possible and biopsies taken, the valve may be impassable. In some cases of longstanding, chronic or healed previous colitis the valve may conversely be atrophic and widely patent, without the usual soft or bulging lips.

Inspecting the terminal ileum

The terminal ileum surface looks granular in air, but underwater the villi float up. The ileal surface is often studded with raised lymphoid follicles resembling small polyps, or these can be aggregated into plaque-like Peyer's patches. Sometimes the ileum is surprisingly colon-like, with a pale shiny surface and visible

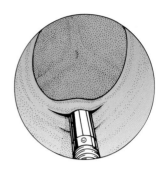

Fig. 6.88 The biopsy forceps can be used to locate, and then pass into, the ileo-cecal valve.

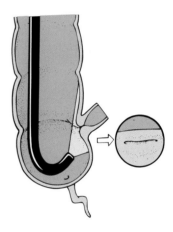

Fig. 6.89 A slit-like valve may only be visible in retroversion.

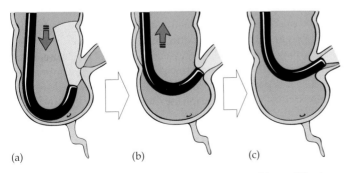

(a) (b) (c)

Fig. 6.90 (a) If necessary retroflex to see the valve … (b)… pull back to impact … (c)… and insufflate and de-angulate to enter the ileum.

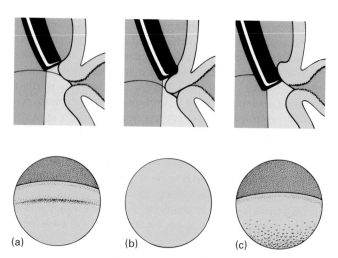

Fig. 6.91 Entering the ileo-cecal valve. (a) Distant view of the valve slit. (b) Pushing in directly impacts against upper lip. (c) Overshooting the valve a little lets the tip angle-in successfully.

submucosal vascular pattern. After colon resection the difference between colon and ileum may be imperceptible because of villus atrophy. Using the dye spray technique—0.1% indigo carmine, 5% methylene blue (which stains) or 1:4 dilution of washable blue (ink)—to highlight the surface detail will rapidly discriminate between the granular or 'sandpaper' appearance of the ileal mucosa and the small circumferential grooves of the colonic surface, which give a 'fingerprint' effect.

The ileum is soft, peristaltic and collapsible compared to the colon, and should be handled more like the duodenum. Rather than attempting forceful insertion, greater distances can be travelled by gentle steering and deflation—so that the intestine collapses over the colonoscope. At each acute bend it is best to deflate a little, hook round, pull back and then steer gently (if necessary almost blindly) around and inward before pulling back again to relocate the direction of view—the 'two steps forward and one step back' approach that applies throughout colonoscopy. When the colonoscope tip is in the ileum, it can often be passed for up to 30–50 cm with care and patience, although this length of intestine may be folded on to only about 20 cm of instrument. Air distension in the small intestine should be kept to a minimum because it is particularly uncomfortable and slow to clear after examination—another reason for routinely using CO_2.

EXAMINATION OF THE COLON

Better views are obtained overall during withdrawal than on insertion, so more painstaking examination is usually performed on the way out. However, in many areas, especially around bends, a different and sometimes much better view is obtained during insertion. For this reason when a perfect view is obtained of a polyp or other lesion during insertion (especially a small one) it is better to deal with it at once (snare, biopsy or image, as appropriate) rather than have the humbling experience of not being able to find the polyp again on the way out and thereby waste time. A convincing example to the endoscopist who doubts this difference between insertion and withdrawal is in the larger number of diverticular orifices seen while inserting around bends (so the colon wall is seen side-on) compared with the relatively few seen on formal examination on the way out.

The colon is shortened and crumpled during insertion and, during withdrawal, the most convoluted or crumpled parts, such as the transverse and sigmoid colon, can spring off the tip at such speed that it is difficult to ensure a complete view. At sharp bends or marked haustrations there may therefore be blind spots during a single withdrawal. Careful scanning and twisting movements should be used in an attempt to survey all parts of each haustral fold or bend, and some may need to be re-examined several times. At a flexure the outside of the bend may be seen on the first pass, but the colonoscope often has to be reinserted and hooked to get a selective view of the other side. Acute bends, including the hepatic and splenic flexures, the sigmoid–descending colon junction and the capacious parts of the cecum and rectum are potential blind spots where the endoscopist needs to take particular care to avoid 'misses' (Fig. 6.92).

Changes of position can help complete inspection. The splenic flexure and descending colon are rapidly filled with air and emptied of fluid by asking the patient to rotate toward the right lateral position. In patients where accuracy is particularly important, such as those with increased risk of polyps or possible bleeding points, it is our policy to rotate them to the right oblique position for inspection of the left colon, then back to the left lateral position again for a better view of the sigmoid colon and rectum.

Single-handed technique comes into its own during inspection on withdrawal. The endoscopist has precise control and the corkscrewing movements made by twisting the shaft are the quickest way of scanning a bend or haustral fold so that he or she can rapidly re-examine a problem area several times. With an assistant, difficulties of communication and coordination make it more difficult to be thorough and accurate.

As well as being obsessional the endoscopist must be honest, reporting not only what is seen but also when the view has been imperfect due to technical difficulty or bad bowel preparation. Even during an ideal examination, the endoscopist probably misses at least 5–10% of the mucosal surface, and in a problematic examination may miss up to 20–30% (although large protuberant lesions are unlikely to be missed).

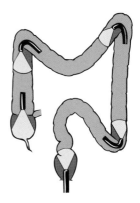

Fig. 6.92 Potential blind spots for colonoscopic visualization.

Localization

Uncertainty in localization is one of the endoscopist's most serious problems, especially during flexible sigmoidoscopy or limited colonoscopy, but even during supposed 'total' or complete colonoscopy. This can lead to mistakes in judging where the instrument has reached and therefore which maneuvers to employ. Endoscopic errors of localization can also be catastrophic if the surgeon is given wrong information around which to plan a resection.

Distance of insertion of the instrument is inaccurate, although sometimes used by inexperienced colonoscopists to express the position of the instrument or of lesions found ('the colonoscope was inserted to 90 cm', 'a polyp was seen at 30 cm', etc.). The elasticity of the colon makes this information meaningless; at 70 cm the instrument may be in the sigmoid colon, in the cecum or anywhere between. On withdrawal, however, providing no adhesions are present and the mesenteric fixations are normal, the colon will shorten and straighten predictably (Fig. 6.93) so that measurement gives approximate localization. On withdrawal, the cecum should be at 70–80 cm, the transverse colon at 60 cm, the splenic flexure at 50 cm, the descending colon at 40 cm and the sigmoid colon at 30 cm (Fig. 6.94). The last two values depend, of course, on the sigmoid colon being straightened. It is sometimes difficult to convince enthusiasts for rigid proctosigmoidoscopy that at 25 cm their instrument may still be in the rectum, whereas the flexible colonoscope (on withdrawal) may be in the proximal sigmoid colon. Equally, it is sometimes possible for the colonoscope to be withdrawn to 55–60 cm when the tip is in the cecum if the colon is mobile.

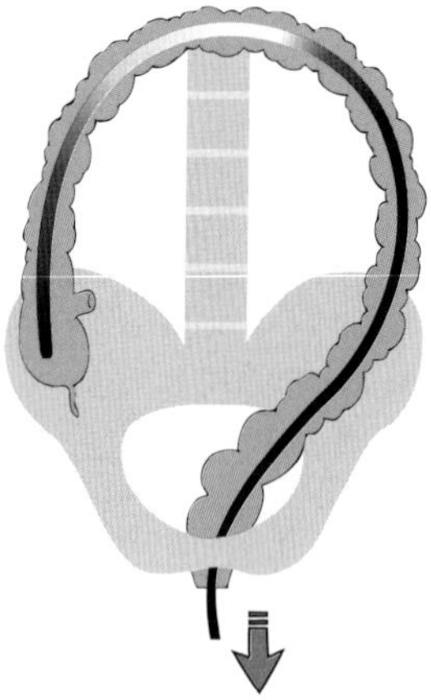

Anatomical localization is inaccurate during insertion. In almost half the cases of a personal series the expert was wrong! In 25%, a persistent loop (alpha or N) caused the endoscopist to judge the tip location to be at the splenic flexure when actually it was at the sigmoid–descending colon junction. In 20%, a mobile splenic flexure pulled down to 40 cm from the anus, causing the endoscopist wrongly to judge the instrument to be at the sigmoid–descending colon junction (see Fig. 6.59). Similar inaccuracies are demonstrated by 3D imager series.

The internal appearances of the colon can be misleading. In the sigmoid and descending colon the haustra and the colonic outline are generally circular (see Fig. 6.11), whereas the longitudinal muscle straps or teniae coli cause the characteristic triangular cross-section often seen in the transverse colon (see Fig. 6.61); the descending colon, however, may look triangular or the transverse colon circular in outline. Visible evidence of extracolonic viscera normally occurs at the hepatic flexure where there is seen to be a bluish/gray indentation from the liver, but a similar appearance may sometimes occur at the splenic flexure or descending colon.

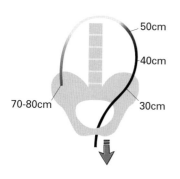

Fig. 6.93 Pulling back the scope shortens the colon.

Fig. 6.94 If the scope is in the cecum at 70–80 cm, other anatomical sites are predictable by measurement.

The combination of an acute bend with sharp haustra and blue coloration is characteristic of the hepatic flexure and is a useful, but not infallible, endoscopic landmark. Pulsation of adjacent arteries is seen in the sigmoid colon (left common iliac artery) and transverse colon (aorta) and sometimes in the ascending colon (right iliac). The *ileo-cecal valve* is the *only* definite anatomical landmark in the colon, but it has been stressed already that it is not always easy to find, and mistaken identification is possible unless the ileum is entered or the orifice visualized.

Fluid levels can be surprisingly useful clues to localization, especially after oral lavage. Just as the radiologist rotates the patient into the right lateral or left lateral position to fill the dependent parts of the colon with barium (Fig. 6.95), the endoscopist (with the patient in the usual left lateral position) knows that the instrument tip is in the descending colon when it enters fluid, and is in the transverse colon when it leaves the fluid for the triangular and air-filled lumen of the transverse colon (see Fig. 6.57). However, a long transverse colon, when it sags down, can also contain a large amount of fluid, so mobile colons are particularly difficult for localization (and everything else).

Transillumination of the abdominal wall by instruments with bright illumination (all video-endoscopes have a bright transillumination facility) can be very helpful if other imaging modalities are not available, but in obese patients may necessitate a darkened room. It should be remembered that the descending colon is so far posterior that no light is usually visible and that the surface marking of the splenic and hepatic flexures is by transillumination through the rib cage posteriorly. Light in the right iliac fossa is suggestive, but not conclusive, that the instrument is in the cecum; similar appearances can be produced if the tip stretches and transilluminates the sigmoid or mid-transverse colon.

Finger indentation, palpation or ballotting can be effective, particularly in the ascending colon or cecum, where close apposition to the abdominal wall should make the impression of a palpating finger easily visible to the endoscopist, unless the patient is obese.

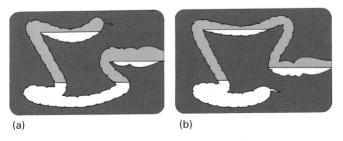

(a) (b)

Fig. 6.95 Barium enema in (a) the left lateral position and (b) the right lateral position.

If in doubt indent in several places and beware the possibility of transmitted forces giving, literally, misleading impressions.

Reporting localization of the instrument tip or lesions found should therefore be made by the endoscopist in broad anatomical terms (e.g. 'the polyp was seen on withdrawing the instrument at 30 cm in the proximal sigmoid colon'), or even omitted altogether so that there is no chance of confusion in the mind of someone unfamiliar with the degree of shortening possible in the colon. Inaccurate localization can occur even when imaging is employed, and the endoscopist usually needs to rely on a combination of assessments—distance inserted; distance after withdrawal and straightening of the shaft; endoscopic (and 3D imager when available) appearances, and possibly visualization of palpating fingers or transillumination. Knowing the pitfalls and being careful should make localization reasonably accurate, but even experienced endoscopists can mistake the sigmoid colon for the splenic flexure, or the splenic flexure for the hepatic flexure, which can be a serious error if localizing a lesion before surgery.

Normal appearances

The colonic mucosa normally shows a generalized fine, ramifying vascular pattern, which can often be seen to be composed of parallel pairs of vessels comprising a venule (larger, bluer) and an arteriole. The veins become particularly prominent in the rectum, notably so in the anal canal if a proctoscope is used to impede venous return, and distend the hemorrhoidal plexus. The vessel pattern in the colon depends on the transparency of the normal colonic epithelium, since the vessels seen are in the submucosa. If the epithelial capillaries are dilated (as may occur after bowel preparation) the vascular pattern may be partly obscured. If hyperemia is marked (as in inflammatory bowel disease) there is no visible pattern. If the epithelial layer is thickened (as in the 'atrophy' of inactive chronic inflammatory disease) the mucosa appears pale and featureless even though biopsies may be essentially normal. The most convincing demonstration of how poorly the endoscopist normally sees the epithelial surface is to spray dye (0.1–2% indigo carmine or 25% dilution of washable blue ink) onto the colonic mucosa. Small irregularities and lymphoid follicles stand out and there is a fine interconnecting pattern of circumferential 'innominate grooves' on the surface into which the dye sinks, providing there is no excess of mucus on the surface.

Prominent vessels should not be thought of as abnormal, and are not likely to be hemangiomatous or variceal, unless they are markedly tortuous or serpentine. Mucosal trauma can occur during insertion of the colonoscope, and red or bloodstained patches may sometimes be seen on withdrawal, especially in the sigmoid or where the looped sigmoid colon has impinged on the upper descending colon. Sometimes it may be wise to irrigate or to take biopsies to ensure that these appearances are not evidence of inflammatory change.

Abnormal appearances

It is not the purpose of this book to cover more than the most obvious points of endoscopic pathology, which are fully covered in the various available atlases of endoscopy. Fortunately for the endoscopist, nearly all colonic abnormalities are either mucosal, with characteristic discoloration, or project into the lumen so that they are easy to see and excise or biopsy.

Submucosal lesions, which may be very difficult to diagnose, include secondary carcinoma, endometriosis, a few large-vessel hemangiomas and dysplastic change in chronic ulcerative colitis. The endoscopist has a poor appreciation of colonic contour due to the nearly fish-eye lens and flat illumination of endoscopes. He or she may also see nothing, or remarkably little compared with the radiologist, of extracolonic communications such as tracks or fistulae. Any experienced endoscopist has also, through bitter experience, learnt humility in visual interpretation and takes care to provide appropriate specimens for pathological opinion as well.

Polyps

The normal colonic mucosa is pale, so submucosal abnormalities are too, such as hamartomatous polyps, lipomas or gas cysts. The *smallest polyps* (of whatever histology) are also pale and those of 1–2 mm diameter may be transparent and invisible except on light reflex or by the dye spray technique. In polyps 3–4 mm in diameter, there may equally be little difference in appearance between a normal mucosal excrescence and a metaplastic, adenomatous or any other type of polyp, although small adenomas are more often red and frequently have a matt-looking or even brain-like ('gyral' or 'sulcal') surface in close-up view. The combination of high-resolution or zoom endoscopes with vital staining (methylene blue) or surface enhancement by dye spraying (indigo carmine) is able to give the endoscopist truly microscopic views, but the clinical impact that this will have is uncertain. Even the smallest polyps are easy to pick out if the patient has been a purgative taker, since the dusky appearance of melanosis coli (often most marked in the right colon) does not stain either polyps, which stand out like pale islands, or the ileo-cecal valve. Flat, sessile, *villous adenomas* may be pale, soft and shiny, but have a rough surface; they are commonest in the rectum.

Larger hyperplastic polyps (7–15 mm in diameter and sessile) can occur in the proximal colon, when they typically appear brown and gelatinous because their surface mucus adsorbs bile.

Apart from lipomas or shiny, worm-like inflammatory polyps, which sometimes have a cap of white slough, all other polyps are usually best removed. Macroscopic differentiation is inaccurate and there is no sure way of anticipating which polyp will prove histologically to be premalignant.

A *malignant polyp* may be obviously irregular, may bleed easily from surface ulceration or be paler, and also firmer than usual to palpation with the biopsy forceps. Such signs of possible malignancy in a stalked polyp warn the endoscopist to electrocoagulate the base thoroughly, to obtain a histological opinion on the stalk and to localize and tattoo the polyp carefully for follow-up and in case subsequent surgery is indicated.

Carcinomas are usually very obvious. They are larger and have a more extensive irregular base; carcinomatous ulcers are uncommon in the colon but look like malignant gastric ulcers. However, *small 'early cancers'* do occur, typically 6–8 cm in diameter with a slightly depressed center. Conditions which can almost exactly mimic malignancy are granulation tissue masses at an anastomosis, larger granulation tissue polyps in chronic ulcerative colitis, and (rarely) the acute stage of an ischemic process. Biopsy evidence should always be obtained, bearing in mind that the pathologist may only be able to report 'dysplastic tissue' since there may not be diagnostic evidence of invasive malignancy in the small pieces presented, which is why either a large-forceps biopsy or snare-loop specimen should be taken whenever possible. Even with standard forceps, a surprisingly large specimen can be taken by the 'avulsion' or 'push biopsy' approach; the instrument is then withdrawn keeping the forceps outside the tip so as not to shear off parts of the tissue by pulling it back through the biopsy channel.

Inflammatory bowel disease

Biopsies must always be taken in any patient with bowel frequency, loose stools or any clinical suspicion of inflammatory disease. 'Microscopic colitis', whether ulcerative or Crohn's, which is clearly abnormal on microscopy, can look absoloutely normal to the endoscopist. The possibly related condition of 'collagenous colitis', a rare cause of unexplained diarrhea due to an extensive 'plate' of collagen under the epithelial surface, also shows normal mucosa visually and the diagnosis can only be made histologically.

Mucosal abnormality can vary enormously in different forms of inflammatory bowel disease. Inflamed mucosa can show the most minute haziness of vascular pattern, slight reddening or tendency to friability. Colonoscopic biopsies unfortunately rarely yield diagnostic granulomas in Crohn's disease, whereas the appearance of multiple, small, flat or volcano-like 'aphthoid' ulcers set in a normal vascular pattern is characteristic. The differential diagnosis of the various specific and non-specific inflammatory disorders may not be easy: infective conditions, ulcerative, ischemic, irradiation and Crohn's colitis can look amazingly similar in the acute stage, although biopsies will usually differentiate between them. The ulcer from a previous rectal biopsy or a solitary ulcer of the rectum can look endoscopically identical to a Crohn's ulcer, whereas tuberculous ulcers are similar but more heaped up, and amebic ulcers are more friable. Ulceration can also occur in chronic ulcerative colitis and ischemic disease but against a background of inflamed mucosa. The endoscopic appearances must be taken together with the clinical context and histological opinion. In the severe or chronic stage it is often impossible for either endoscopist or pathologist to be categoric in differential diagnosis.

Unexplained rectal bleeding, anemia or occult blood loss

Blood loss or anemia is a common reason for undertaking colonoscopy. Although colonoscopy gives an impressive yield of radiologically missed cancers and polyps, 50–60% of patients will show no obvious abnormality, which raises the specter of whether anything has been missed.

Hemorrhoids can be seen with the colonoscope (by retroversion in the rectum if necessary), but a proctoscope should be used for a proper view and the endoscope tip can be inserted within it to show the patient or take video-prints at 'video-proctoscopy'.

Hemangiomas are rare, but they can assume any appearance from massive and obvious submucosal discoloration with huge serpentine vessels to telangiectases or minute solitary nevi, which could easily be missed in folds or bends.

Angiodysplasias are rare and mainly occur in the cecum or ascending colon, but also in the small intestine. They have variable appearances, may be solitary or multiple (often two or three) and are always bright red, but they can be small vascular plaques, spidery telangiectases or even a 1–2 mm dot lesion.

Pain and 'pain mapping'

Irritable bowel symptoms are probably the commonest single reason for referral. Functional bowel disturbance in an otherwise normal colon can take many forms, and 'spastic colon' pain may present with equally variable referred-pain radiation patterns—to the right or left loin, back or even into the thighs. An occasionally useful and very simple colonoscopic procedure is to map the pain experienced during distension at different sites in the colon produced by inflating a small balloon taped alongside the tip of the colonoscope (Fig. 6.96). A child's balloon, finger-cot or the cut-off finger of a rubber glove is bound with fine thread

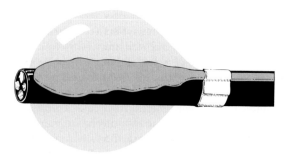

Fig. 6.96 Balloon for pain mapping taped behind the colonoscope tip.

at the end of a catheter. The bound neck of the balloon is taped to the junction of the colonoscope shaft and bending section—placing the balloon at the tip can obscure the view—and two or three additional tapes secure it along the shaft. With a three-way tap and a 50 mL Luer-fitting syringe it is easy to inflate and deflate the balloon in representative sites during withdrawal of the colonoscope. The balloon should not be inflated above 200 mL volume in the proximal colon and 100 mL distally, otherwise mucosal stretch damage will occur. Because of the variability in colon size, making a quantitative relationship between the volume inflated and the pain experienced in different patients is unpredictable, but some patients with irritable bowel syndrome/spastic colon are notably hypersensitive to even 25 mL distension in the sigmoid colon. At each inflation site ask the patient about the quality and site of any pain experienced, and use this to map out referred-pain radiation sites and their correlation with the patient's 'usual' symptoms.

STOMAS

If a finger can be inserted into any stoma, a standard or pediatric colonoscope will also pass without trouble, but a pediatric gastroscope can be substituted if necessary. It is quite normal for the stoma to change to an unhealthy looking cyanotic color and even for there to be a little local bleeding, but no harm ensues.

Through an ileostomy, the distal 20 cm of ileum are easily examined (ideally with a pediatric colonoscope) but further insertion depends on whether adhesions have formed. As in the sigmoid colon, the secret of passage through the small intestine is to pull the instrument back repeatedly as each bend is reached, which convolutes the intestine onto the instrument and straightens out the next short segment; thus even though only 30–40 cm of instrument can be inserted, as much as 50–100 cm of intestine may be seen.

Colostomy patients are usually easy to examine since the sigmoid colon will usually have been removed. The colon can be remarkably long, however, and full bowel preparation is essential. Colostomy washouts are less effective. The first few centimeters through the abdominal wall and proximal to the colostomy are sometimes awkward to negotiate and to examine, partly because of the continual escape of insufflated air. If there is a loop colostomy the afferent and efferent (proximal and distal) sides can be examined.

Pelvic ileo-anal pouches are easy to examine with a standard instrument. Limited examination of an ileal conduit is possible, using a pediatric endoscope (colonoscope or gastroscope).

PEDIATRIC COLONOSCOPY

Pediatric colonoscopy, from neonatal to 3–5 years of age, is best performed with a thinner (1 cm), preferably 'floppy', pediatric colonoscope. In older children, depending on physique, adult colonoscopes can be used, and for teenagers they are mandatory. The infant anus will accept an adult little finger and so will take an endoscope of the same size. The neonatal sphincter first requires gentle dilation over a minute or two, using any small smooth tube (such as a nasogastric tube or a ballpoint pen cover). The main advantage of a purpose-built pediatric colonoscope is more the extra flexibility or 'softness' of its shaft than its small diameter, because it is easy with stiffer adult colonoscopes to overstretch the mobile and elastic loops of a child's colon. It is generally a mistake to use a pediatric gastroscope for anything but a very limited inspection because it is much stiffer. An adult 13–15 mm colonoscope, although usable, is nonetheless too clumsy to be ideal in the colon of a small child—reminiscent of driving a large articulated truck through small alleyways—uncomfortable for all concerned.

Who should perform pediatric colonoscopy is a matter of local judgment. Few pediatricians do enough colonoscopy to become really dextrous. If complete colonoscopy is required it may often be best for examination to be by a skilled adult endoscopist, with the pediatrician present.

Bowel preparation in children is usually very effective. Pleasant-tasting oral solutions such as senna syrup or magnesium citrate are best tolerated. A saline enema will cleanse most of the colon of a baby.

General anesthesia is frequently used, although children of any age can be colonoscoped without general anesthesia providing that the endoscopist is experienced. Reasonable intravenous medication is used, but a pediatrician with experience of resuscitation must be present as a safeguard. A suitable oral sedative premedication (such as antihistamine or pethidine) can be useful so that a particularly anxious child is relaxed before the procedure. A small dose of intravenous (IV) benzodiazepine (Diazemuls® 2–5 mg or midazolam 1–3 mg) is usually combined with a larger dose of pethidine (meperidine) 25–50 mg IV, slowly titrated according to response and body weight. When the child is somnolent and tolerates digital examination easily, the rest of the colonoscopy will be equally well tolerated. Neonates may sometimes be more safely examined with no sedation at all.

PERIOPERATIVE COLONOSCOPY

Exsanguinating bleeding is rare, but is an indication for perioperative colonoscopy; 'on-table' cecostomy lavage preparation is used to give a reasonable view. Otherwise perioperative colonoscopy is normally only justified if attempts at colonoscopy have failed in a patient with known polyps, where the small intestine is to be examined in a patient with continued blood loss, or where the colon proximal to a constricting neoplasm is to be inspected to exclude synchronous lesions.

Oral lavage or full colonoscopy bowel preparation must be used in non-obstructed patients as most standard preoperative preparation regimens leave solid fecal residue. If the bowel has been completely obstructed, it is possible to perform on-table lavage through a temporary cecostomy tube or through a purse-string colotomy proximal to the obstructing lesion. During perioperative colonoscopy, overinsufflation of air can fill the small intestine and leave the surgeon with an unmanageable tangle of distended loops. This can be avoided if the endoscopist uses CO_2 insufflation instead of air, or if the surgeon places a clamp on the terminal ileum and the endoscopist aspirates carefully on withdrawal.

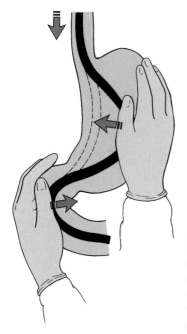

To examine the small intestine at laparotomy, if an enteroscope is not available a long (preferably variable) colonoscope can be used—either perorally or through an intestinal incision; 70 cm of instrument is required to reach either the ligament of Treitz perorally or the cecum peranally. It helps if the surgeon either mobilizes or manually supports the fixed part of the duodenum (see Fig. 6.97) if the colonoscope is passed orally. The small intestine must be very gently handled on the endoscope to avoid local trauma or postoperative problems. It is also important to insufflate as little as possible. Clamps are sequentially placed on each segment of small intestine after it has been evacuated. The surgeon inspects the transilluminated intestine from outside (with the room lights turned off) while the endoscopist inspects the inside. The surgeon marks any lesion to be resected with a stitch while the endoscopist can perform conventional snare polypectomies as appropriate. A major source of confusion tends to be the artefactual submucosal hemorrhages that occur from handling the small intestine.

Fig. 6.97 Perioperative straightening of the stomach and duodenum.

INSTRUMENT TROUBLE-SHOOTING

The functionality of all instrument controls should be checked before examination, because they can be difficult to spot or tedious to remedy during it. Colonoscopy can be difficult enough without adding problems in instrument performance.

Vision

Check the illumination and clarity of view beforehand. Is the light source functioning properly and the brightness control turned up? Is the view crisp or is there debris on the lens or light-bundle lenses that may need washing or polishing off? Colonic mucus and debris can be solidified by the protein-denaturing effects of strong antiseptics such as glutaraldehyde. Use a hand-lens to inspect the tip optics closely and to help with local cleaning.

Air

If there is no insufflation from the tip, check the light source—is the air pump switched on, are the umbilical and water-bottle connections pushed in fully and the water bottle screwed on? Is the rubber O-ring in place on the water-bottle connection? Is the air/water valve in good condition and seated properly and the CO_2 valve in position (where relevant), since it will otherwise allow air leakage. As already mentioned, proper air insufflation is difficult to assess by bubbling under water compared with the obvious efficacy of blowing up a rubber glove or balloon held over the scope tip. It is easy to miss the fact that there is inadequate air flow during an examination, which then becomes technically difficult and the colon apparently 'hypercontractile' because it collapses continually and inflates with difficulty. A great deal of wasted time can be avoided by noticing this defect before starting, or by withdrawing the scope at an early stage to check and rectify the problem.

Organic debris and mucus can cause poor insufflation, tending to reflux back up the air channel due to the positive pressure within the colon. A particular culprit is the small, angled air/water pipe at the tip of the instrument. A single plug or an accretion of layers of proteinaceous material can solidify within the metal pipe, especially after glutaraldehyde exposure. Paradoxically, the units with the greatest 'air-blockage' problems are often those with the highest cleaning standards, where full antisepsis is rigorously employed. The problem can be minimized by careful water-flushing of the air channel for at least 30–40 seconds immediately after each examination. Preferably, this should be achieved with a single-channel flushing device, since any adaptor that flushes both the air and water channels simultaneously will simply by-pass an absolute or partial blockage in one channel without this being apparent. Using enzyme detergents is also very effective in the cleaning process, including domestic non-foaming versions for endoscope washing machines.

Special 'channel flushing devices' allowing direct pressure syringing are available from some manufacturers. A messy alternative is to activate the regular air valve, put a finger over the water-bottle port on the umbilical to avoid leakage, and then to syringe through the air-input channel at the end of the umbilical using a suitable syringe attachment, such as a micropipette tip cut to size. If the air channel cannot be unblocked during the process of an examination a simple dodge is to empty the water bottle, then to activate the water valve to achieve air insufflation (use the water syringe attachment if lens washing is needed).

The tiny angled metal 'air pipe' of some instruments' tips can need direct attack if there is an air blockage problem. First try probing its slit-like opening, or even water-injecting this using a fine-gauge intravenous needle. If this proves ineffective it is possible, as a last resort, to remove the air nozzle altogether, which usually means returning the instrument to the manufacturer's service department. A skilled technician can remove, clean and reinsert the air pipe very easily. Other manufacturers have removed this problem by introducing ingeniously designed removable tips, allowing more thorough channel cleaning between examinations.

Water-wash failure

Failure of the water system is unusual (other than from an empty water-bottle), because mucus or debris do not reflux back into the water system as easily as they do into the empty air channel. Nonetheless, particles of rubber O-ring or other matter can become lodged in the water system. They should be quickly cleared by water-syringing with a micropipette tip into the small hose that normally lies underwater within the water bottle—remembering to press the water valve simultaneously to allow flow.

Suction failure

The suction valve itself can become obstructed, which should be obvious on careful inspection. Particulate debris can also block the suction channel. If in the shaft, this can be dislodged by water-syringing through the biopsy port. Removing the suction valve and covering the opening on the control head with a finger is a quick way of improving suction pressure and can result in rapid clearance of the whole system (as when sucking polyp specimens). Applying the sucker tube directly to the suction-channel opening can also be effective in clearing particulate debris. As a final resort the whole suction system can be cleared by retrograde-syringing using a 50 mL bladder syringe to wash through tubing attached to the suction port on the umbilical. Push the suction valve and also cover the biopsy port during this procedure to avoid unpleasant (refluxed) surprises.

FURTHER READING

General sources

Rex DK. Colonoscopy. *Gastrointest Endosc Clin North Am* 2000; 10: 135–60.

Sivak MV Jr, ed. *Gastroenterologic Endoscopy*, 2nd edn. Philadelphia: WB Saunders, 1995.

Waye JD, Rex DK., Williams CB. *Colonoscopy.* Oxford: Blackwell Publishing, 2003.

Preparation, medication and management

Axon AT, Beilenhoff U, Bramble MG *et al.* Variant Creutzfeldt–Jakob disease (vCJD) and gastrointestinal endoscopy. *Endoscopy*; 2001; 33: 1070–80.

Bell GD. Premedication, preparation, and surveillance. *Endoscopy* 2002; 34: 2–12.

Eckardt VF, Kanzier G, Willems D, Eckardt AJ, Bernhard G. Colonoscopy without premedication versus barium enema: a comparison of patient discomfort. *Gastrointest Endosc* 1996; 44: 177–180.

Fleischer D. Monitoring the patient receiving conscious sedation for gastrointestinal endoscopy: issues and guidelines. *Gastrointest Endosc* 1989; 35: 262–5.

Hussein AMJ, Bartram CI, Williams CB. Carbon dioxide insufflation for more comfortable colonoscopy. *Gastrointest Endosc* 1984; 30: 68–70.

Kim LS, Koch J, Yee J, Halvorsen R, Cello JP, Rockey DC. Comparison of patients' experiences during imaging tests of the colon. *Gastrointest Endosc* 2001; 54(1): 67–74.

Martin JP, Sexton BF, Saunders BP, Atkin WS. Inhaled patient-administered nitrous oxide/oxygen mixture does not impair driving ability when used as analgesia during screening flexible sigmoidoscopy. *Gastrointest Endosc* 2000; 51: 701–703.

Saunders BP, Fukumoto M, Halligan S Patient-administered nitrous oxide/oxygen inhalation provides effective sedation and analgesia for colonoscopy. *Gastrointest Endosc* 1994; 40: 418–21.

Stevenson GW, Wilson JA, Wilkinson J, Norman G, Goodacre RL. Pain following colonoscopy: elimination with carbon dioxide. *Gastrointest Endosc* 1992; 38: 564–7.

Techniques and indications

Arigbabu AO, Badejo OA, Akinola DO. Colonoscopy in the emergency treatment of colonic volvulus in Nigeria. *Dis Colon Rectum* 1985; 28: 795–8.

Bosset de V, Froehlich F, Rey JP *et al*. Do explicit appropriateness criteria enhance the diagnostic yield of colonoscopy? *Endoscopy* 2002; 34: 360–8.

Brooker JC, Saunders BP, Shah SG, Williams CB. A new variable stiffness colonoscope makes colonoscopy easier: a randomised controlled trial. *Gut* 2000; 46: 801–805.

Friedman S, Rubin PH, Bodian C, Goldstein E, Harpaz N, Present DH. Screening and surveillance colonoscopy in chronic Crohn's colitis. *Gastroenterology* 2001; 120: 820–6.

Harris GJ, Senagore AJ, Lavery IC, Fazio VW. The management of neoplastic colorectal obstruction with colonic endolumenal stenting devices. *Am J Surg* 2001; 181: 499–506.

Hixson LJ, Fennerty MB, Sampliner RE, Garewal HS. Prospective blinded trial of colonoscopic miss-rate of large colorectal polyps. *Gastrointest Endosc* 1991; 37: 125–7.

Jensen DM, Machicado GA. Diagnosis and treatment of severe hematochezia. The role of urgent colonoscopy after purge. *Gastroenterol* 1988; 95: 1569–74.

Kalvaria L, Kottler RE, Marks IN. The role of colonoscopy in the diagnosis of tuberculosis. *J Clin Gastroenterol* 1988; 10(5): 516–23.

Kingham JGC, Levison DA, Ball JA, Dawson AM. Microscopic colitis—a cause of chronic watery diarrhoea. *Br Med J* 1982; 285: 1601–4.

Nelson DB. Technical assessment of direct colonoscopy screening: procedural success, safety, and feasibility. *Gastrointest Endosc Clin North Am* 2002; 12: 77–84.

Rex DK, Cutler CS, Lemmel GT, Rahmani EY, Clark DW, Helper DJ, Lehman GA, Mark DG. Colonoscopic miss rates of adenomas determined by back-to-back colonoscopies. *Gastroenterol* 1997; 112: 24–28.

Rex DK, Bond JH, Feld AD. Medical-legal risks of incident cancers after clearing colonoscopy. *Am J Gastroenterol* 2001; 96: 952–7.

Rex DK. Rationale for colonoscopy screening and estimated effectiveness in clinical practice. *Gastrointest Endosc Clin North Am* 2002; 12: 65–75.

Rutgeerts P, Wang TH, Llorens PS, Zuccaro G, Jr. Gastrointestinal endoscopy and the patient with a risk of bleeding disorder. *Gastrointest Endosc* 1999; 49: 134–6.

Shah SG, Brooker JC, Williams CB, Thapar C, Saunders BP. Effect of magnetic endoscope imaging on colonoscopy performance: a randomised controlled trial. *Lancet* 2000; 356: 1718–22.

Shah SG, Brooker JC, Williams CB, Thapar C, Suzuki N, Saunders BP. The variable stiffness colonoscope: assessment of efficacy by magnetic endoscope imaging. *Gastrointest Endosc* 2002; 56: 195–201.

Swarbrick ET, Bat L, Hegarty JE, Dawson AM, Williams CB. Site of pain from the irritable bowel. *Lancet* 1980; 443: 446.

Waye JD, Bashkoff E. Total colonoscopy: is it always possible. *Gastrointest Endosc* 1991; 37: 152–4.

Waye JD, Yessayan SA, Lewis BS, Fabry TL. The technique of abdominal pressure in total colonoscopy. *Gastrointest Endosc* 1991; 37: 147–51.

Webb WA. Colonoscoping the 'difficult colon'. *Am Surg* 1991; 57: 178–82.

Wexner SD, Garbus JE, Singh JJ. A prospective analysis of 13,580 colono-scopies. Reevaluation of credentialing guidelines. *Surg Endosc* 2002; 15: 251–61.

Winawer SJ, Stewart ET, Zauber AG *et al.* A comparison of colonoscopy and double-contrast barium enema for surveillance after polypec-tomy. National Polyp Study Work Group. *N Eng J Med* 2000; 342(24): 1766–72.

Villavicencio RT, Rex DK, Rahmani E. Efficacy and complications of argon plasma coagulation for hematochezia related to radiation proc-topathy. *Gastrointest Endoscopy* 2002; 70–4.

Hazards and complications

Kavin RM, Sinicrope F, Esker AH. Management of perforation of the colon at colonoscopy. *Am J Gastroenterol* 1992; 87: 161–7.

Macrae FA, Tan KG, Williams CB. Towards safer colonoscopy: a report on the complications of 5000 diagnostic or therapeutic colonoscopies. *Gut* 1981; 24: 376–83.

Rockey DC, Weber JR, Wright TL, Wall SD. Splenic injury following colonoscopy. *Gastrointest Endosc* 1990; 36: 306–9.

Tran DQ, Rosen L, Kim R, Riether RD, Stasik JJ, Khubchandani IT. Actual colonoscopy: what are the risks of perforation? *Am Surg* 2001; 67(9): 845–7.

Waye JD, Kahn O, Auerbach ME. Complications of colonoscopy and flex-ible sigmoidoscopy. *Gastrointest Endosc Clin North Am* 1996; 343–77.

7 Therapeutic Colonoscopy

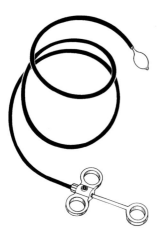

Fig. 7.1 Use one commercial snare type for familiarity.

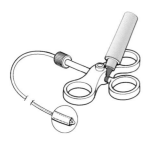

Fig. 7.2 Mark the handle when the loop is fully closed.

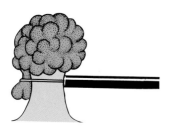

Fig. 7.3 Polyp tissue can be trapped in the snare, reducing its efficiency.

EQUIPMENT

The equipment requirements for endoscopic polypectomy are few, and in many ways the fewer the better. It adds significantly to safety to be completely familiar with one electrosurgical unit, and only a few accessories, since from this familiarity it becomes easy to recognize when polypectomy is going right and when it is not.

Snare loops

Be familiar with the type of snare used. For anyone doing a limited number of polypectomies it is advisable for endoscopist and assistant to be familiar with one or two snare types only. Several makes of snare loop are available, and different handle characteristics and wire thicknesses greatly affect control of polypectomy. Single-use snares have the advantage of always being in good condition and predictable. Reusable snare loops and wires can become deformed or may be reassembled into non-standard plastic outer tubes. Many endoscopists prefer to use a standard larger snare (2.5 cm diameter) and a 'mini-snare' (1 cm diameter for smaller polyps) and specialist spiked, barbed or stiffer snares are available for sessile polyps (Fig. 7.1). Various configurations of snare loop or variations of handle are available, but are mainly a matter of personal preference.

With any snare there are several points that should be checked *before* starting polypectomy:
1 *Mark the snare handle with a pencil or indelible pen at the point that the snare is just closed* to the tip of the outer sheath (Fig. 7.2). This is arguably the single most important safety factor in polypectomy. It allows the assistant to stop snare closure before the wire closes too far into the tube and there is danger of a smaller stalk being cut off by 'cheese-wiring' mechanically without adequate electrocoagulation; it also warns if the stalk is larger than apparent or head tissue has become entrapped (Fig. 7.3). Marking can also, but less conveniently, be performed *after* insertion by looking for the moment when the wire emerges from the snare catheter. Many snare handles have marker numbers moulded in or printed on, but making a physical mark is safer—because the mark proves that the point of wire closure has been exactly checked, and it is easier to see.

2 *A smooth 'feel' is essential for safety*; the snare handle and wire should open and close easily so that the endoscopist (or assistant) has an accurate idea of what is happening if the snare loop is out of view behind the polyp or its stalk. A reusable snare inner wire that has been bent in use or cleaning and no longer moves freely within its plastic outer sheath is hazardous and should be discarded.

3 *Snare-wire thickness* greatly affects the speed of electrocoagulation and transection. Most loops are made of relatively thick wire so that there is little risk of cheese-wiring unintentionally and there is a larger contact area which favors good local coagulation rather than electrocutting. Some single-use snares have thin wire loops and need a lower current setting or care in closure to avoid cutting too rapidly, before full coagulation of stalk vessels. Be careful if using a new snare type.

4 *Squeeze pressure* is very important, especially when snaring large polyps. There should be a 15 mm closure of the wire loop into the snare outer tube before use (Fig. 7.4a). This ensures that the loop will squeeze the stalk tightly even if the plastic outer sheath crumples slightly under pressure, a particular problem with large stalks (see p. 174). If squeeze pressure is inadequate (Fig. 7.4b) the final cut may have to rely entirely on using high-power electrical cutting and may not coagulate the central stalk vessels enough, with potentially disastrous (bleeding) consequences. If the loop closes too far (Fig. 7.4c) cheese-wiring can occur before electrocoagulation is applied. This can also result in bleeding.

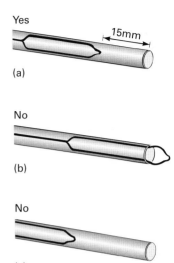

Fig. 7.4 (a) Snare closed 15 mm is right; (b) wire too loose; (c) wire too tight.

Other devices

Hot biopsy forceps are used to destroy small polyps up to 5 mm in diameter and even for electrocoagulating telangiectases or angiodysplasia, if argon plasma coagulation (APC) is unavailable (see pp. 13–14, 183).

Polyp retrieval is possible with a variety of accessories—memory metal Dormia-type basket, nylon net, multi-prong grasping forceps and a polyp suction trap. These can all be useful, especially for multiple or piecemeal-removed polyp specimens, but a snare loop is often adequate for picking up a severed polyp and saves time in changing accessories.

Injection needles are invaluable for saline or epinephrine (adrenaline) injection, whether for elevation of sessile polyps, to prevent or arrest bleeding or to tattoo a polypectomy site.

Dye-spray cannulas allow visualization or surface detail interpretation of small or flat polyps, and the margins of sessile polyps, although dye can (perhaps more easily) also be syringed in without a cannula.

Clipping or nylon-loop placement devices have an occasional invaluable place, either to deal with postpolypectomy bleeding or to prevent it. The metal clips available are too short-jawed to be useful for the thick stalks most at risk, and the nylon loop is difficult to place over a larger head. Either can be placed on the residual stalk when there is bleeding or increased risk of it—as in patients with a bleeding diathesis or on anticoagulants or similar medication. Ideally both a loop (EndoLoop®, Olympus) and a clipping device should be available, pre-primed in case of a sudden bleed. They are relatively fiddly to assemble in a crisis, so practice is desirable. The single-use clipping device (Quick Clip®, Olympus) overcomes this problem, a first gentle squeeze opening-up the clip and a further (forcible) squeeze closing it.

Principles of polyp electrosurgery

Electrosurgical or diathermy currents cause heat, coagulating local blood vessels—especially the large ones. The coagulated tissue also becomes easier to transect with the snare wire, but this is of secondary importance. Heat is generated in tissue by the passage of electricity (electrons), the flow of which causes collisions between intracellular ions and release of heat energy in the process (Fig. 7.5). The high-frequency or 'radio-frequency' electric current, alternates in direction at up to a million times per second (10^6 c/s, 1000 kc/s or 1 MHz) (Fig. 7.6).

There is no 'shock' or pain at such high frequencies, because there is no time for muscle and nerve membrane depolarization before the current alternates again and therefore no muscle contraction or afferent nerve impulse. Electrosurgical current is therefore not felt by the patient and there is equally no danger to cardiac muscle. This is in contrast to low-frequency household currents, which shock because they alternate only 50–60 times per second (50 c/s) (Fig. 7.7). At the low power used in polypectomy, even the unlikely possibility of a direct thermal burn to the skin of a patient or operator is surprising but trivial, and actual burns are very rare because the local heat would cause a strong protest long before actual damage occurred. The only real danger from electrosurgical currents is their heating effect on the bowel wall at the site of electrocoagulation.

Modern cardiac pacemakers are unaffected at the relatively low power used for endoscopic electrosurgery. An additional safety factor is that the electrosurgical current passage between the polypectomy site in the abdomen and patient plate (usually on the thigh) is reasonably remote from the pacemaker. If in doubt consult a competent cardiologist.

Coagulating and cutting currents

Cutting current has an uninterrupted (and so high-power) waveform of relatively low voltage spikes (Fig. 7.8). The interrupted current flow excites the air molecules into a charged 'ionic cloud', visible as high-temperature sparking that vaporizes the surface cell

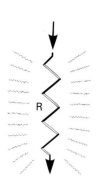

Fig. 7.5 Heat is generated by electricity (electrons) passing through resistance (R)—in this case tissue.

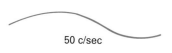

10⁶ c/s

Fig. 7.6 An electrosurgical current alternates 1 000 000 times per second, producing heat but no shock.

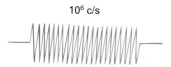

50 c/sec

Fig. 7.7 A household current alternates 50–60 times per second, producing heat and shock.

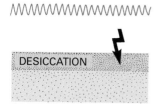

DESICCATION

Fig. 7.8 Cutting current—continuous (high-power) low-voltage pulses cannot pass desiccated tissue.

layer to steam. Because it is low voltage, however, cut current is less able to traverse desiccated tissue and to heat deeply. 'Auto-cut' intelligent electrosurgical units automatically adjust power output to match the resistance of the tissue being heated in order to produce a predictable rate of transection.

Coagulating current has intermittent higher-voltage spikes with intervening 'off periods', which last for about 80% of the time (Fig. 7.9). The higher voltage allows a deeper spread of current flow across desiccating tissue, whereas the off periods reduce (except at high power settings) the tendency for gas ionization, sparking and local tissue destruction.

Blended current combines both waveforms (Fig. 7.10), some units providing the ability to select blends with relatively greater 'cut' than 'coag' characteristics. The differences between the various makes of electrosurgical unit suggest that the output characteristics are more complex than this brief summary suggests, some appearing to provide more effective hemostasis than others. When changing from one unit to another it is therefore essential to be cautious, to start with low power settings. If possible, try out the unit on a small lesion or the periphery of a larger one, rather than entering the 'big-time' unrehearsed and then regretting it.

Current density

Tissue heats because of its high electrical resistance, typically around 100 ohms, although resistance varies according to the particular tissue (fat conducts poorly and so heats little); water loss (desiccation) during heating increases resistance and the drying tissue is also mechanically harder to transect. If electric current is allowed to spread out and flow through a large area of tissue, the overall resistance and heating effect falls (Fig. 7.11). To obtain effective electrocoagulation, the flow of current must be restricted through the smallest possible area of tissue—the principle of 'current density' (Fig. 7.12). This principle is basic to all forms of electrosurgery and explains why no noticeable heat is generated at the broad area of skin contact with the patient 'return plate', whereas intense heat occurs in the closed snare loop (Fig. 7.13). Even a relatively small area of contact between the buttock or thigh and patient plate is adequate, and extra moisture or electrode jelly is unnecessary at the power used for endoscopic polypectomy.

The essential in polypectomy is to coagulate the core of the polyp stalk, with its plexus of arteries and veins, *before* transection. Closing the snare loop both stops the blood flow ('coaptation') and tends to concentrate the current to flow through and heat-coagulate the core (Fig. 7.14). The tightness of the loop is critical, since the area through which the current is concentrated (current density) decreases as the square of snare closure (πr^2), thus causing a square law relationship between snare closure and increasing current

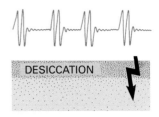

Fig. 7.9 Coagulating current—intermittent high-voltage pulses can pass desiccated tissue.

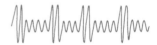

Fig. 7.10 Blended current combines the characteristics of both cutting and coagulating currents.

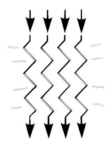

Fig. 7.11 Current flows more easily through larger areas of tissue resistance and so produces little heat.

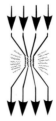

Fig. 7.12 Current density results from constricting tissue and greatly increases heating.

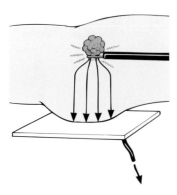

Fig. 7.13 Heating occurs at the closed snare but not at the plate.

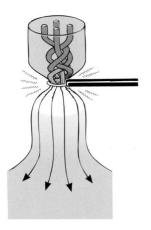

Fig. 7.14 The whole plexus of stalk vessels must be electro-coagulated before section.

density. The heat produced increases as the square of current density, so heating increases as the *cube* of snare closure (i.e. a slight increase of snare closure on a polyp stalk greatly increases the heat produced). Conversely, the fact that the closed snare loop is the narrowest part of the stalk means that the base of the stalk and the bowel wall should scarcely heat at all, which explains the rarity of bowel perforations during or after stalked polypectomy. Contact pressure between snare wire and polyp surface and thickness of snare wire (thinner wire, greater heating) are additional factors, with a square law relationship between contact area and heat produced.

Heating of a polyp stalk increases proportionately to increase in power setting on the unit dial (Fig. 7.15) and it also increases directly as time passes (ignoring complicating features such as heat dissipation) (Fig. 7.16).

Closure of the snare loop is the most important variable, because of the cubed increase of heat production as the snare closes (Fig. 7.17). If the snare is too loose it will hardly heat the tissue at all; if too tight it will heat the tissue too fast. The soft stalk of a small polyp should, therefore, coagulate rapidly; a larger stalk, being less compressible, requires a slightly higher power setting and more time before visible tissue coagulation occurs. Visually it can be difficult to be absolutely sure of the diameter and consistency of the stalk, since the view may be poor and the wide-angle lens distortion can be confusing. The 'feel' of the stalk may also be inaccurate, especially with snares having a thin and compressible plastic sheath, which can result in the snare handle being 'closed' when the stalk is actually inadequately narrowed (Fig. 7.18). It is to allow for this 'crumpling' under pressure that a check for loop closure 15 mm within the sheath is so important before snaring a large polyp with a new snare-type. Equally, it is to allow time to react to what is happening that the recommendation is to perform polypectomy using coagulating current only, and at a low power setting (corresponding to only 15–25 W). Only occasionally should it be necessary to increase the power if no visible coagulation has occurred; extra time will usually do the job. The 'auto cut' setting of some electrosurgical

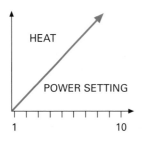

Fig. 7.15 Heat produced is directly proportional to power …

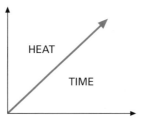

Fig. 7.16 … and directly proportional to time …

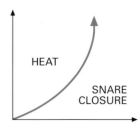

Fig. 7.17 … but increases as the *cube* of snare closure.

units adjusts output automatically for appropriate heating during snaring.

'Slow cook' is the essential principle of polypectomy, so as to electrocoagulate an adequate length of stalk tissue before section. There should be visible whitening as the protein denatures, with swelling or even steam as the stalk tissue boils. Remember that some tissue necrosis effect may extend beyond the zone of obvious electrocoagulation whitening, which is a particular consideration in avoiding mucosal ulceration and secondary bleeds after 'hot biopsy' in particular. However, if all the water boils off, electrons will no longer flow through the desiccated tissue of a polyp stalk and the wire may have to be pulled through mechanically—in principle a somewhat risky thing to do, because thick-walled vessels are usually the last part to sever. Inevitably it takes a little time at the safer lower current settings to heat the tissue but, if this takes more than 30–40 seconds, the risk of heat dissipation at a distance (and damage to the bowel wall) increases and it may be more realistic to increase the power setting to speed things up. The maximum power setting used should be equivalent to no more than 30–50 W.

Thick stalks (1 cm or more in diameter) are more difficult to coagulate, with a risk of inadequate central vascular electrocoagulation, particularly if the stalk is firm and relatively non-compressible and the vessels within it are large and thick-walled. A higher power setting may be needed to start electrocoagulation peripherally or tight snaring may be needed to start electrocoagulation, with a rapid increase of heating and the unfortunate effect that, as the snare starts to transect and close down through the stalk, the heat produced increases very dramatically. This results in electrocutting of the central core, precisely the part that needs slow and controlled coagulation. Additional factors such as current leakage from 'contralateral' contact points may complicate things further and are discussed later.

If no coagulation is occurring in a large polyp stalk check:
- *Are the circuitry and connections correct?*
- *Is the snare handle properly assembled and closed?*
- *Has the stalk been correctly snared—or the head trapped out of sight (see Fig. 7.3)?*
- *If the stalk is very thick consider epinephrine injection (Fig. 7.19), have nylon loop or clip ready.*
- *Can the snare loop be repositioned higher up the stalk where it is narrower?*

If there is any fear of complications or the operator is inexperienced, this may be the moment to disengage the snare and leave the procedure to someone else (see below for how to disengage a 'stuck' snare).

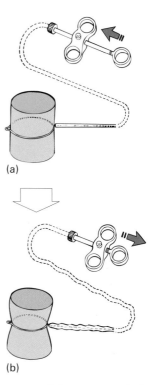

(a)

(b)

Fig. 7.18 When snaring a thick stalk (a) the plastic sheath may crumple before closure is adequate (b).

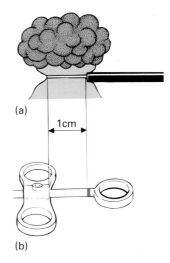

(a)

1cm

(b)

Fig. 7.19 (a) Thick stalks can bleed—think of pre-injection. (b) The distance to the closure mark indicates the stalk size.

POLYPECTOMY

Stalked polyps

Even an expert can have difficulty snaring some polyps. A beginner, unskilled in handling the colonoscope, can miss seeing them or get inadequate views of a larger polyp, resulting in unsafe or incomplete snaring.

The following steps and points should help guarantee safe and effective polypectomy:

1 *Check and mark the snare.* An overenthusiastic but inexperienced assistant can 'cheese-wire' through the polyp stalk before adequate electrocoagulation by closing the snare handle completely or too forcibly. This is particularly likely if the snare wire is thin or the polyp stalk is small. The mark on the snare handle indicates the point at which the tip of the snare loop has closed down to the end of the outer sheath. This can be done visually beforehand or when the snare is already within the colon (see Fig. 7.2). When a thick stalk is snared the mark gives a useful approximate measure of its size and a warning that there may be problems (Fig. 7.19b).

2 *Get to know the electrosurgical unit.* When first using an electrosurgical unit, start with the lowest dial setting and use initial bursts of 2–3 seconds at each increased setting. Discover the lowest dial setting (usually 2.5–3) that causes visible controlled electrocoagulation in the smallest stalk.

3 *Develop a standard routine for polypectomy* and always follow it. Check the connections, plate position and the electrosurgical unit setting before each polypectomy. Make sure that the foot pedal is in a convenient position, preferably where it can be felt with the foot without having to look down to search for it at the critical moment after the polyp is grasped. A polyp can suddenly shift if the patient moves or coughs.

4 *Use the closed snare outer sheath to assess the base or stalk mobility* of larger polyps. Visual assessment of the stalk size can be difficult due to the distorting effect of the wide-angle endoscope lens. Comparing the stalk size to the 2 mm width of the protruded plastic snare sheath and pushing it around to assess length and mobility can be invaluable—warning that extra power and/or longer time will be needed for transection.

5 *Open the snare loop within the instrument channel* when snaring small or average-sized polyps. This avoids the need to manipulate the snare handle when the loop emerges from the endoscope. Lassoing the polyp head efficiently takes practice. It is usually best to have the loop fully open, and then to maneuver only with the instrument controls or shaft, so that the snare loop is placed over the polyp head almost entirely by manipulation of the endoscope. It may help to open the snare in the colon beyond the polyp, and then to pull the colonoscope slowly back until the polyp head comes into the field of view and into the open loop. Alternatively, the loop can be pushed backwards over a difficult polyp head (Fig. 7.20), or placed to one side or other of the polyp head and then swung over it by appropriate movements of the instrument. Effective rotatable snares are now available and may have a useful place for 'problem' polypectomies, where access is difficult.

6 *Optimize the view and position of the polyp* before becoming committed, especially if the polypectomy looks as though it may be awkward—which is often only apparent after trying to place the loop over the polyp head. A change of patient position can improve the view of the stalk and rotation of the colonoscope shaft to exit the forceps or snare in a better position, at the bottom right of the field of view, means that the view is not lost during polypectomy (Fig. 7.21).

7 *Snare the polyp and push the snare sheath against the stalk* (the 'push' technique), which ensures that closing the loop will tighten it exactly at the same point. If the sheath is not pushed against the stalk, loop closure by the assistant will tend to move or even pull the wire off the polyp (Fig. 7.22) unless the endoscopist simultaneously advances the sheath (the 'pull' technique). If there is any doubt that the snare is properly over the polyp head, try shaking the snare or opening and closing the loop repeatedly to help it slip down around the stalk. Vigorous angulation of the colonoscope tip in the relevant direction may help, even if this means losing an ideal view.

8 *Close the snare loop gently,* to the mark or by feel, until it is closed. Snare closure occurs ideally near the top of the stalk at its narrowest part, leaving a short segment of normal tissue to help pathological interpretation (Fig. 7.23). Initial snare closure should be gentle; the loop may be in the wrong place and once the wire has cut into polyp tissue it may be difficult to release and reposition it. With longer stalks, especially if there is any suspicion of malignancy, it may be possible and desirable to snare lower down to increase the chance of resecting all invasive tissue in the stalk.

9 *If the snare loop is stuck in the wrong position* or if it becomes apparent that the polyp cannot be safely transected, releasing the snare loop is made easier by lifting it up over the polyp head and pushing forcibly inward—with the whole colonoscope if necessary (Fig. 7.24). If ever the loop is completely trapped in a polyp, a second small-diameter instrument (gastroscope or pediatric colonoscope) can be inserted alongside the first scope and the biopsy forceps used to coax the wire free. Remember that it is always possible (depending on type) either to dismantle the snare or to sacrifice it by cutting it with wire cutters, withdrawing the colonoscope and leaving the loop *in situ*. Either the polyp head will fall off or another attempt can be made with a new snare or,

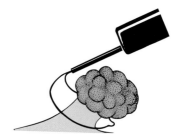

Fig. 7.20 Backward snaring is sometimes useful.

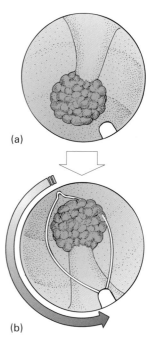

(a)

(b)

Fig. 7.21 (a) Bad position for snare placement? (b) Rotate the instrument to get a better working position and view.

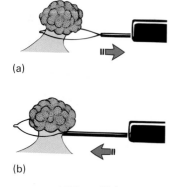

(a)

(b)

Fig. 7.22 (a) To avoid the snare pulling off during closure (b) push the loop against the stalk before closing.

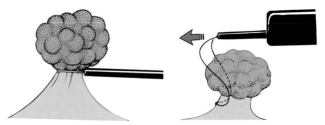

Fig. 7.23 Snare at the narrowest part of the stalk.

Fig. 7.24 To disengage a trapped snare, push it upstream over the polyp head.

if necessary, a different endoscopist. It is never necessary to be 'committed' to a polypectomy just because it has been started.

10 *Electrocoagulate using a low-power coagulating current* (15 W or dial setting 2.5–3) with the snare loop kept *gently* closed to 'neck' the tissue and create favorable circumstances for electrocoagulation. Apply the current continuously for 5–10 seconds at a time, watching for visible swelling or whitening. Once the stalk or base below the snare is visibly coagulating, squeeze the handle more tightly while continuing electrocoagulation, and transection will start.

11 *Watch where the polyp head falls*, or time may be wasted looking for it. If it is lost, look for any fluid, which indicates the dependent side of the colon, where the severed polyp head is likely to have fallen. If none is visible, squirt in some water with a syringe and watch where it flows. If the water simply refluxes back over the lens, the polyp will also be distal to the instrument tip and the endoscope will need to be withdrawn to find the specimen.

12 *Retrieval of the specimen* may be with the snare or one of the retrieval devices (such as the multi-wire 'memory metal' Dormia basket (Fig. 7.25) or the nylon Roth net (Fig. 7.26). Suctioning the polyp onto the tip of the endoscope may mean having to withdraw and reinsert the instrument because the reduced view on withdrawal usually compromises examination of the remaining colon. In the presence of numerous polyps it may be pragmatic to snare/transect some specimens of medium size to allow them to be aspirated and so save time. Suction pressure and likelihood

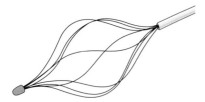

Fig. 7.25 Multi-wire 'memory metal' basket.

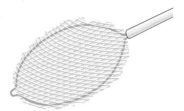

Fig. 7.26 Nylon polyp retrieval net.

of successfully aspirating the specimen is increased by removing the suction valve (the narrowest part of the suction channel), occluding the opening with a finger and waiting—some seconds if necessary—until the polyp compresses and shoots through. Smaller polyps or portions up to 6–7 mm can be aspirated through the channel into a filtered suction trap (Fig. 7.27) or, more cheaply, onto a gauze placed over the suction connector on the light guide plug at the end of the umbilical (Fig. 7.28).

Small polyps

Tiny polyps are just as awkward to snare as larger ones, and can be difficult to retrieve, even using the filtered suction trap. There has therefore been a tendency for some endoscopists to ignore small polyps or to describe them as 'hyperplastic', wrongly inferring that small polyps have no neoplastic potential. On biopsy, 70% of such small polyps prove to be adenomas, and only around 20% of those in the colon (as opposed to the rectum) are hyperplastic. Small polyps in the colon should therefore be destroyed or removed on sight. The best method of doing this is a matter of debate, for surprisingly large (1–2 unit) secondary bleeds can occur 1–12 days after removal or electrodestruction of a 1–2 mm polyp.

Snare or 'cold snare'?

Mini-snares are more convenient for snaring small polyps. After snaring, retrieval by aspiration into a suction trap is a convenient way of managing many polyps 5–7 mm in diameter. Larger polyps are unlikely to be able to be aspirated through the instrument channel unless fragmented by the snare or in the suction

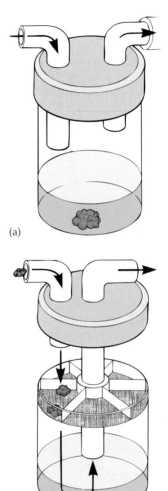

(a)

(b)

Fig. 7.27 (a) An old-style mucus trap. (b) A filtered polyp suction trap.

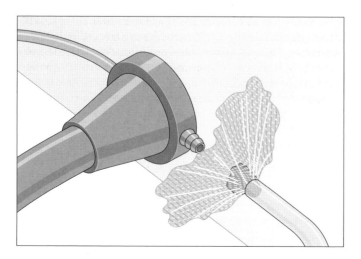

Fig. 7.28 Gauze inserted over suction connector for polyp retrieval.

process. Snaring has the advantage over hot-biopsy of squeezing the polyp base, so reducing the area and depth of electrocoagulation damage to the remaining mucosa and underlying blood vessels. Some endoscopists go further and advocate 'cold snaring' without electrocoagulation, particularly in the proximal colon, physically pulling through the base of the small snared polyp in order to avoid any risk of heat ulceration and delayed bleeds.

Snaring very small polyps can be technically difficult and the specimens are not infrequently lost. Use of the filtered suction trap for retrieval is a significant improvement over the older mucus aspiration trap (designed for bronchoscopy or neonatal care), because each specimen is trapped in a separate numbered compartment and the incorporated filter prevents specimen loss even if excess fluid has to be aspirated. Putting a gauze in the suction line is cheaper for single polyps.

'Hot biopsy'

Hot biopsy forceps are a quick and effective way of destroying the smallest (1–4 mm) polyps (Fig. 7.29a), in spite of some bad press due to occasional bleeding complications. They have the particular virtue of yielding over 95% of interpretable histology—compared with the frequent specimen losses after snaring. Histology is potentially important in managing a patient because the total number of adenomas is the most important predictor of future risk of neoplasm, so should influence advice on follow-up (see below). The hot biopsy forceps are only different from conventional diagnostic forceps in having a plastic insulation outer sheath and a handle with electrical connection to the electrosurgical unit, the circuit connecting back via a patient plate, just as for polypectomy. The same low-power 'coag' setting (15–25 W or equivalent) is used as for snaring a small polyp. The specimen taken (often only 10–20% of the whole polyp) is protected from current flow within the forceps jaws, so is unheated (unless by thermal conduction resulting from over-lengthy current application). By contrast, provided that the technique is properly performed, within 1–2 seconds there is intense local heating of the tissues and blood supply beneath, resulting in surprisingly dramatic but superficial ulceration—which heals over the next two weeks.

Safe hot biopsy depends on localizing the heating effect by careful attention to details of technique:

1 *Select only a suitably small polyp*—and don't be too proud to abandon hot biopsy and change to (mini-) snaring if the polyp proves to be bigger than expected.

2 *Only the apex of the small polyp is grasped* in the jaws of the hot-biopsy forceps (Fig. 7.29b), deliberately *not* forcing them into the colon surface below, as is normal in taking a mucosal biopsy.

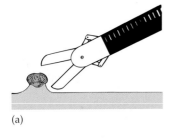

(a)

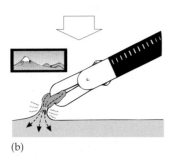

(b)

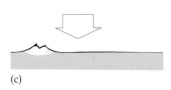

(c)

Fig. 7.29 (a) Hot biopsy forceps grasp the small polyp and pull up... (b)...then coagulate until there is 'snow on Mount Fuji'... (c)...pull off the biopsy sample, leaving the coagulated polyp base.

3 *'Tent up' the polyp onto a 'pseudo-pedicle'* (like a small mountain) by colonoscope angulation or by withdrawing the forceps slightly. This elevation is made possible because of the loose stroma of submucosa over the underlying colon wall (analogous to that of the skin over the back of the hand)—although hazardous in the thin proximal colon.

4 *Ensure that the black insulating plastic of the forceps is visible*, so that the metal parts of the jaws do not contact the endoscope.

5 *Apply coagulating current for a maximum of 2–3 seconds.* Because the pseudo-pedicle is the narrowest part, local current density should result in almost immediate heating and electrocoagulation. The extent of coagulation is visible as whitening, but this should ideally spread only halfway down the 'mountain'—the 'Mount Fuji effect' (Fig. 7.29b). Further spread is unnecessary, as even normal-looking tissue is heated and will subsequently become necrotic.

6 *Pull off the biopsy* in the knowledge that, even if some of the head is left uncoagulated, the basal tissue and blood vessels will have been destroyed and it will slough off.

Polyps over 5 mm in diameter are not suitable for hot biopsy removal. Either the base will be broader than the area of contact of the forceps (so only a small burn will result at the surface of the polyp) (Fig. 7.30) or, more dangerously, the current will fan out from the point of contact of the hot biopsy forceps (Fig. 7.31) (heating tissue at a distance, invisibly causing necrosis). Coagulating for too long or attempting to destroy over-large polyps with the hot biopsy technique therefore risks causing a deep ulcer with the chance of delayed hemorrhage or even of full-thickness heating and perforation (both risks especially great in the proximal colon). So, if a polyp proves to be too large for rapid and localized visible electrocoagulation, *stop*, take the biopsy, and remove the rest of the tissue by conventional snare polypectomy.

PROBLEM POLYPS

Sessile polyps

It is difficult to achieve 'current density' for localized heating when snaring a sessile or broad-based polyp. This is why removal of large sessile polyps (Fig. 7.32a) or broad-stalked polyps presents problems for the endoscopist and why piecemeal removal can be the safer option. It is also for this reason that 'auto-cut' electrosurgical units may be an advance, because they provide the high power needed to start transection but reduce it rapidly to safer levels thereafter. Fortunately, many so-called 'sessile' polyps up to 10–15 mm in diameter are simply 'semi-pedunculated' or, if 'broad-based', can be pulled up by the snare onto an adequate and compressible pseudo-stalk. Alternatively

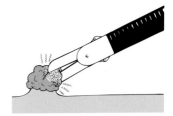

Fig. 7.30 Local burning at the forceps means the polyp is too large for hot biopsy.

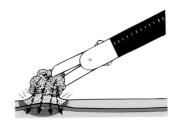

Fig. 7.31 Current fanning out from the point of contact will heat (invisibly) at a distance, risking delayed bleeding or perforation in polyps too large for hot biopsy.

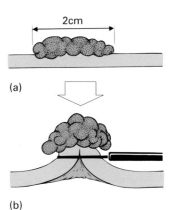

Fig. 7.32 (a) Sessile polyps can be risky to snare in one portion... (b)...because 'tenting' results.

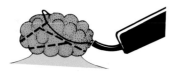

Fig. 7.33 Piecemeal removal is safer (although less satisfactory for the pathologist).

submucosal injection can be used to elevate the polyp tissue before snaring (see below).

Move the closed snare to and fro as a measure of safety having snared all or part of a sessile polyp; if the mucosa moves, but not the bowel wall, there is no danger. If the colon moves with the snare, the full thickness of the wall has been 'tented' dangerously (Fig. 7.32b) and the snare should be repositioned to take only a smaller part. If the base of a protuberant polyp is over 1.5 cm in diameter, with no stalk, the safe course is to take the head piecemeal in a number of bits (Fig. 7.33); each bit can be cut through with no risk of full-thickness burns and little risk of bleeding, since the vessels of the head are much smaller than those in the stalk. With the submucosal injection technique described below, however, it may be possible to remove flat sessile polyps up to 1.5–2 cm in diameter in a single specimen, and much larger ones piecemeal.

Injection polypectomy

Submucosal saline injection elevates sessile polyps for easier removal, a technique common in proctology and originally described for colonoscopic use in 1973. Injection has become a frequent routine, initially with the intention of obtaining small sessile polyps (flat adenomas) as a single histopathological specimen (Fig. 7.34). 'Injection polypectomy' or endoscopic mucosal resection (EMR), as it is often called, can also be invaluable for the removal of much larger polyps, having the double advantage of creating a bloodless plane for transection and a 'safety cushion' of engorged submucosal stroma that protects the bowel wall from heat damage. Injection can also be with normal saline (0.9%) or 1 : 10 000 epinephrine in 0.9% saline, but this absorbs in 2–3 minutes, so snaring needs to be reasonably quick. To make the injected bleb last longer, a hypertonic solution can be injected (2 N saline, 20% dextrose or hyaluronic acid have all been used, with or without epinephrine). Some experts add a few drops of methylene blue when making up the solution, the blue showing up the extent of the submucosal bleb. With a 10 mL syringe attached, the sclerotherapy needle is either jabbed tangentially into the mucosal surface adjacent to the polyp or directly through the polyp tissue. A relatively slow, low-pressure injection gives time, if necessary, to withdraw the needle slightly until a submucosal bleb is seen to be forming. The 'plane of separation' in the submucosa for successful injection is surprisingly superficial and the tendency is to inject too deep, although there is no hazard involved should the needle or solution pass into the peritoneum (or the peritoneal cavity). An injection of 1–3 mL should be enough to raise the submucosa below a small polyp for immediate snaring, but 20–30 mL may be needed for larger polyps.

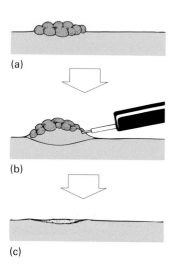

(a)

(b)

(c)

Fig. 7.34 Injection polypectomy. (a) A small sessile polyp ... (b)... is elevated by submucosal saline injection ... (c)... and snared off in one piece.

Make the first injection proximal to a large sessile polyp, so that the raised bleb of tissue does not obscure the view. Make each subsequent injection into the edge of the preceding bleb (Fig. 7.35) or inject directly through the polyp surface (providing the polyp is thin enough for the needle to reach the submucosa below). Up to 30 mL total injection volume may be needed to raise a 4–5 cm sessile polyp.

Failure of injection to elevate a sessile polyp (the 'non-lifting sign') suggests malignancy, the lesion being fixed by invasion into deeper layers. If non-lifting occurs, take no risks in attempting total removal but wait for histology and consider assessment by endoscopic ultrasound or other form of scanning. Surgery is likely to be necessary.

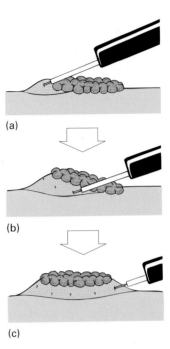

(a)

(b)

(c)

Fig. 7.35 (a) First inject *proximally* to a larger sessile polyp... (b)... then around the periphery ... (c)... to elevate it completely before snaring.

Large sessile polyps

Even very large sessile polyps can often be removed endoscopically, but this should be a matter of expert opinion and clinical judgment. As a 'rule of thumb' it has been suggested that sessile polyps occupying more than one-third of the colon circumference, or involving two haustral folds, are too big for safe endoscopic removal. The endoscopic approach is the obvious one in a patient who is a bad operative risk and is prepared to accept repeated endoscopy. In a younger patient, or if colonoscopy is technically difficult, it may be better to consider surgery or laparoscopy. Sessile polyps up to 10 cm or more in diameter can be tackled, but only if the endoscopist is sufficiently experienced and the patient appreciates the potential hazards involved, with likely need for multiple examinations.

At the first endoscopic session attempt complete piecemeal removal, because scarring will make subsequent attempts at submucosal injection less likely to succeed. Injection is a significant help in safe debulking, but the main requirements are endoscopic dexterity, patience and sufficient time; piecemeal removal of a very large polyp can take up to 30–40 minutes. The basal remnants, after most of the polyp has been snared, are easily and safely destroyed with argon plasma coagulation (APC) (Fig. 7.36). Before finishing, a submucosal India ink tattoo is left adjacent, because further sessions will be needed to check the site for recurrent polyp tissue, or in case histological assessment indicates surgery.

A pediatric scope can be used in retroversion to pre-inject or snare the proximal part of a polyp if it proves to be difficult to see or target. Other tricks are useful on occasion. Standard polypectomy snares sometimes slip off the moist and domed pre-injected area, and a 'barbed snare' is available, the barbs hooking into the tissue satisfactorily. A stiffer thin monofilament snare can similarly be effective for cutting into the polyp (bleeding is not a significant risk in sessile polyps). A 'needle-knife' has been used by some to

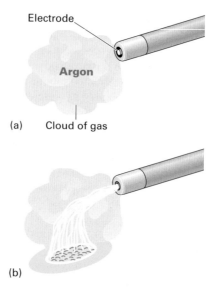

Electrode

Argon

(a)   Cloud of gas

(b)

Fig. 7.36 (a) Argon plasma coagulation (APC) catheter with internal wire electrode emits argon gas cloud. (b) Activating electrosurgical unit ionizes gas, conducting electrocoagulating current to tissue (and patient plate).

pre-cut around the injected and raised polyp margin, allowing the snare to grip it better. A spike-tipped snare can fix the tip of the snare into the mucosal surface at an appropriate point, making opening and control of the loop easier; the tip of a standard snare can be similarly anchored by (very brief) electrocoagulation of the tip, fixing it into mucosa. More complex polypectomy approaches have been tried (but not generally used) such as employing a two-channel instrument with a grasper passed through the opened snare. The grasper is used to elevate the polyp; the snare is then pushed down over the raised polyp, closed and polypectomy performed.

Pain during sessile polypectomy, unless due to overinsufflation, is a warning that full-thickness heating of the bowel wall is occurring, activating peritoneal pain receptors. Fortunately pain is felt before there is any risk of serious damage—another reason for avoiding routine heavy sedation or anesthesia. If pain occurs and deflation does *not* stop it (it is easy to be overenthusiastic with the air button when trying to keep a good view during a problematic polypectomy), the procedure should be abandoned until another session at least 3 weeks later—when healing should have occurred and the area can be properly assessed.

Large rectal polyps

Large sessile polyps up to 12 cm from the anal verge are extraperitoneal (below the peritoneal reflexion) and may sometimes be better removed by local proctological techniques, which often produce a single large specimen for optimum histology—rather than the chaos of fragments resulting from endoscopic piece-meal snaring. Anesthesia allows anal dilation and a two-handed approach for injection and scissor-excision, with the potential to ligature or suture bleeding points if necessary. A failed endo-scopic attempt to remove such rectal polyps forms scar tissue, which hinders submucosal epinephrine injection and excision by the proctologist, so the endoscopist's decision to refer should be made on the basis of visual assessment alone. Only 1:200 000 epinephrine solution is used in the rectum (compared with 1: 10 000 solution in the colon) because very large volumes may be needed and there is risk of communication to the systemic circulation, and danger of serious cardiac dysrhythmias. Sessile polyps more than 12 cm above the anal margin can alternatively be reached with a Buess operating sigmoidoscope (transanal microsurgery or TEMS), where this is available, but will more often be managed by the flexible endoscopist using injection and piecemeal removal with argon plasma coagulation.

Smaller rectal polyps close to the anal canal can be snared in retrover-sion after local anesthetic injection, unless the polyp is very small and quick to snare (perhaps by 'cold-snaring'). The distal 3–5 cm of the rectal ampulla is otherwise difficult to visualize properly and is also richly supplied with sensory nerves, a heat burn caus-ing the same pain as it would on exterior skin.

Large stalked polyps

The 'large' size of a polyp is sometimes an illusion because the visual judgment of size is made relative to the diameter of the colon lumen. Proximal colon and cecal polyps thus tend to be *larger* than they look at first sight. In the narrowed lumen of diver-ticular disease, polyps that appear large may prove on snaring to be significantly *smaller.*

In snaring a large stalk, extra electrocoagulation is needed to minimize the increased chance of bleeding from the relatively large plexus of stalk vessels, and extra care (and time) should be taken to optimize things before starting:

1 *Check that an epinephrine-filled injection cannula can be rapidly available* in case of bleeding, and probably a clipping device and nylon EndoLoop® as well.

2 *Palpate and move the stalk* around using the closed snare to judge its diameter, length and mobility.

3 *Get the best view possible;* if necessary rotate the endoscope or change patient position (Figs 7.21 and 7.37).

4 *Place the snare optimally on the narrowest part of the stalk* to ensure maximal current density.

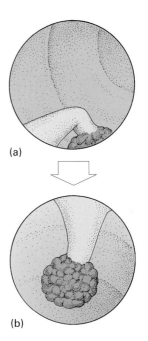

(a)

(b)

Fig. 7.37 (a) Bad view of a polyp? (b) Change the patient's position to let gravity help.

5 *Consider 'pre-snaring' lower down the stalk* in order to extend the zone of electrocoagulation. Squeeze the snare *gently* for this preliminary stalk heating, so that transection doesn't occur and the snare is easy to release and replace higher up the stalk for conventional polypectomy.

6 *Electrocoagulate the stalk* for longer than usual, until visible swelling and whitening indicate that it is safe to start transection.

7 *Consider using a higher than usual current setting*, especially if, in the process of transection, the core desiccates and the snare will not make the final cut. Resist the urge to 'pull through' the snare. The thickest arteries are the last to sever, so it is safer to raise the current setting further and let current heating help to make the cut.

In snaring large stalked polyps, complications, especially bleeding, need to be anticipated (and so often avoided). Large polyps inevitably have larger, thicker-walled and more numerous feeding vessels. Epinephrine and an injection catheter should be available for immediate use if required, and it is highly desirable to have EndoLoop® and clipping devices also. By employing a careful 'slow cook' polypectomy technique, the precautionary methods described below and the crisis-control (or prevention) accessories, we have experienced no serious immediate hemorrhage after polypectomy for many years. Delayed bleeds, however, do continue to happen unpredictably.

Contralateral burns are essentially a 'non-problem.' During snaring of a large stalked polyp, the head will flop about, inevitably touching the bowel wall in several places. 'Leak' currents flow at each point of contact, which results in inefficient heating of the stalk (Fig. 7.38) and the possibility of a contralateral burn—often out of the field of view. The burn hazard is mainly theoretical and the possibility can be avoided by moving the snared polyp head around during coagulation, which ensures that no one point gets all the heat. Alternatively make sure that the area of contact between the head and the opposite wall is large, so that resistance is low and heating insignificant.

During a difficult polypectomy try to keep a view of the snared stalk, especially if only part of the polyp can be seen, and ensure that adequate visible coagulation occurs *below* the snare loop before transection. (If leak currents do flow up the stalk to a contact point at the head, electrocoagulation can occur primarily *above* the snare (Fig. 7.39) and bleeding could result from inadequately coagulated vessels in the lower part of the stalk.)

If there is any doubt about stalk electrocoagulation when the polyp head has severed and if the stalk remnant shows too little visible electrocoagulation whitening, or visible vessels at the center, it may be wise to 'post-snare' lower down, squeezing the stalk gently and electrocoagulating further (without transection) before reopening and removing the loop.

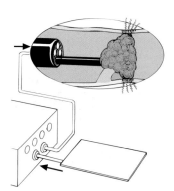

Fig. 7.38 'Leak' current can result in contralateral burns.

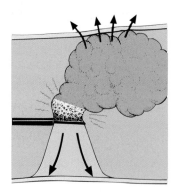

Fig. 7.39 A large area of contact reduces the risk of contralateral burn, but also reduces current flow and heat coagulation in the lower stalk.

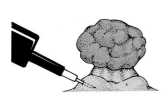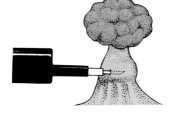

Fig. 7.40 (a) Inject broad-stalked polyps with epinephrine before snaring to avoid bleeding.

(b) For long-stalked polyps with a risk of bleeding inject sclerosant and epinephrine.

Stalk preinjection with epinephrine before snaring makes immediate bleeding unlikely (Fig. 7.40a). Epinephrine (1–10 mL 1:10 000 dilution in 0.9–1.8% (1 N or 2 N) saline) is injected at one or more sites into the base of the polyp and causes visible blanching from vessel contraction within a minute or so. The endoscopist sees blanching and swelling of the stalk and finally mauve coloration of the ischemic head. Transection through the upper part of the stalk or above the injected area can then be made in the certain knowledge that there will be no bleeding.

Nylon EndoLoops® or metal clipping devices are particularly relevant to large-stalked polyps or, in patients on anticoagulants or aspirin, as a way of strangulating the remaining stalk. The most certain method for larger stalks is the nylon self-retaining EndoLoop® (Fig. 7.41). The loop is usually placed on the stalk remnant *after* polypectomy, because the floppy loop is difficult to maneuver over a polyp head of 2 cm or more. For smaller stalks, one or more metal clips can be placed easily before or after snaring. Clips are particularly useful in controlling local bleeding after sessile polypectomy, when there is no stalk on which to close a loop.

Recovery of polypectomy specimens

Extraction of large polyps (3 cm or more) through the anal sphincters can be difficult. The polyp will often fragment if excessive traction is needed on the snare or retrieval grasper, although a multi-wire Dormia basket or polyp-retrieval nylon net should avoid this. Once at the anus ask the patient to bear down 'as if to pass wind' in order to relax the sphincters; at the same time gentle traction is applied to produce the polyp (cover the perineal area to avoid explosive surprises!). If withdrawal fails in the left lateral position, ask the patient to squat on the floor or sit on a commode seat, which is more physiological and (with traction maintained on the retrieval device) rapid expulsion of the polyp invariably results—compensating for any embarrassment about the maneuver. Alternatively, a split overtube can be inserted into the rectum over the colonoscope, the polyp pulled

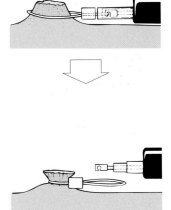
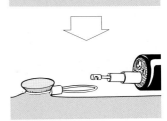

Fig. 7.41 (a) A nylon self-retaining loop can be placed over a large stalk …(b)… and its self-retaining cuff tightened; (c)… and the loop unhooked leaving the stalk strangulated.

into the end of the tube and the whole assembly removed together. A large rigid proctoscope and tissue-grasping or sponge-holding forceps can be similarly used, pulling out the polyp and instrument together.

Multiple polyp recovery

Ninety per cent of adenoma patients have only one or two polyps and it is very uncommon to find more than five. Some multiple polyps (hyperplastic, Peutz–Jeghers, juvenile, lymphoid, lipomatous or inflammatory) are non-neoplastic, so that it may sometimes be preferable to await results of standard biopsies before undertaking heroic numbers of polypectomies, which are probably more risky than the lesions themselves. In the rare circumstance that a patient has six or more obvious adenomas, it is essential to examine the whole colon before snaring, to be certain that multiple other smaller polyps are not present (with the possibility of a diagnosis of familial adenomatous polyposis, or FAP). Looking for tiny reflective nodules in the 'light reflex' off the transparent mucosal surface shows up polyps down to 1 mm in diameter that are invisible to direct vision. Melanosis coli also shows up tiny non-pigmented polyps or lymphoid follicles very well.

Dye spray ('chromoscopy') enhances the view of fine detail, almost to dissecting microscope level. The principle is to use a spray of surface dye (0.1–0.2% indigo carmine solution or 10% dilution of non-permanent blue fountain-pen ink) (see p. 156), which shows up any small polyps down to under 0.5 mm in size, seen as pale islands on a blue background. Dye can be applied using a dye-spray catheter, usually while withdrawing the scope. An easier way is to use 5 mL of dye in an air-filled 20–30 mL syringe inserted into the rubber biopsy valve of the scope, which takes only a few seconds to dye a short segment of colon without using a catheter. Silicone-emulsion anti-bubble solution can be added to the dye to avoid small bubbles, which can look confusingly like tiny polyps. Histology of any polyp seen is essential for certainty because lymphoid follicles can resemble adenomas to the untutored eye (although usually dimpled or 'umbilicated' at their centers).

Retrieval of multiple polyps for histology is a matter of compromise in order to avoid needing to reinsert the colonoscope multiple times. In practice retrieval can be facilitated by use of accessories such as the multi-wire basket or polyp-retrieval net, which are able to retrieve up to three to five moderately large polyps at a time, whereas only one or two polyps can be picked up in the polypectomy snare. Any smaller polyps are either destroyed by hot biopsy or snared and then aspirated into a filtered polyp suction trap or into a gauze placed in the suction line (see Fig. 7.27). A 'wash-out' technique is a rarely needed compromise after the snare removal of large numbers of non-neoplastic polyps (Peutz–Jeghers syndrome, juvenile or inflammatory polyposis). On first presentation of some such patients, as many as 60–100 such polyps may need removal, although their histology is of secondary interest since there is little or no malignant potential. The multiple snared polyps are first retrieved to the descending or sigmoid colon, the colonoscope is then passed to the splenic flexure and 500 mL of warm tapwater is syringe-injected through the instrument channel. The proximal colon is air-insufflated until the patient feels some distension and, just before the colonoscope is withdrawn from the anus, a disposable or phosphate enema can be injected through the endoscope. This ensures evacuation and passage of most of the polyps or polyp fragments into a commode within a few minutes.

Inflammatory polyps of 1 cm or larger should be removed since sporadic adenomas can occur in colitis patients. Most postinflammatory polyps, sometimes called pseudo-polyps, appear as small shiny worm-like tags of healthy and non-neoplastic tissue after the healing of previous severe colitis of any kind. They can be ignored or, if in doubt, a few biopsies can be taken to confirm their trivial nature. Larger postinflammatory polyps have a tendency to bleed and there may be difficulty in distinguishing them from adenomas since they can be composed of granulation tissue or disorganized tissue remarkably similar to that of a hamartomatous (juvenile) polyp. These larger polyps can bleed surprisingly after snaring, partly because they tend to have soft bases that 'cheese-wire' through too quickly compared with the more muscular pedicle of other polyps, but also because they may be very vascular. Any broad-based or sessile polyp, and especially any raised plaque occurring after longstanding ulcerative or Crohn's colitis must be treated with suspicion, since it may represent a so-called 'DALM' (dysplasia-associated lesion or mass), the most visible part of a 'field change' of high-grade dysplasia. With such dubious lesions, take mucosal biopsies around the base before snaring to discount this possibility.

Malignant polyps

Malignancy is suspected if a polyp is irregular, ulcerated, firm to palpation or thick-stalked. Firmness to palpation with the snare tube is probably the best single discriminant. If malignancy is possible, it is important to be certain that transection has been made low down the stalk (to allow the pathologist a proper assessment) and to ensure that any invasion within the stalk has been removed, although without risking perforation. The endoscopist should report, on the basis of multiple vertical cross-sections, whether or not the polyp has been completely removed. If necessary an early repeat examination can be made, preferably within two weeks while there is visible healing ulceration to

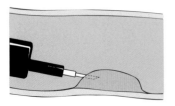

Fig. 7.42 A 1 mL India ink tattoo marks a polypectomy site permanently.

indicate the polypectomy site (and allow biopsy and tattooing). Because of the possibility of malignancy, each polyp is ideally retrieved and identified separately on an anatomical 'colon map' in a biopsy book kept available in each endoscopy room. It is inadequate to say that a polyp was removed at '70 cm from the anus' because this might equallly represent the mid-sigmoid colon or cecum.

Tattooing marks the site of any suspicious or partially removed polyp, whether for follow-up or possible surgery. Sterile diluted India ink is injected intramucosally (Fig. 7.42). A volume of 1 mL adjacent to the polypectomy site is sufficient for endoscopic follow-up, but four quadrantic injections ensure visibility if surgery is a possibility. The problem of ink leakage and 'black-out' of the endoscopic view can be avoided by first injecting a small saline bleb submucosally, then changing syringes so that the 1 mL India ink aliquot enters the bleb. The carbon particles of India ink remain in the submucosa for many years (probably for life), easily visible to the endoscopist as a blue-gray stain. If pre-sterilized India ink is unavailable, a syringe-mounted bacterial filter is said to be effective. As a reasonable last resort *non*-waterproof India ink can be diluted and used instead; select the type used for water-color painting or brushing and not calligraphic pen ink, which contains noxious materials such as shellac or solvents and can cause inflammation or peritoneal pain.

Adequate removal of a malignant polyp is a recurrent problem, especially if the histopathologist's report of malignancy comes as a surprise to the endoscopist. Although non-specific features of large size, induration or irregular surface may arouse suspicion, the macroscopic appearance of a malignant polyp can be unremarkable. The clinician or endoscopist is then faced with a dilemma but, happily, one that can usually be resolved in favor of conservatism (rather than surgery), certainly for pedunculated polyps. If the cancer is histologically 'well' or 'averagely well' differentiated, with a margin of 1 mm or more between the limit of invasion and the transection line, and also assuming that endoscopic removal also appeared complete, surgery is *not* recommended. The likelihood of there being residual local tumor or resectable lymph node involvement under these circumstances is extremely small (ignoring the even more remote, but ever present, possibility of unresectable distant metastases), whereas the 1% mortality of surgery in older patients is immediate.

Surgery is indicated for a malignant polyp:
• that is sessile
• when invasion extends histologically within 1 mm of the resection line
• when the carcinoma is poorly differentiated (anaplastic)— and so more likely to metastasize.

Under these circumstances the likelihood of involved lymph nodes is significant and most would favor operation, *unless* the patient is considered to be a poor surgical risk. Clinical judgment is involved, balancing risks and clinical factors in the interests of long-term survival. Review of the histological slides is essential and a second opinion from a specialist histopathologist may be indicated. The opinion of the patient or the patient's family should be sought and may also swing the decision. If there is any doubt, it may be difficult not to operate in a young patient, mainly for emotional reasons and for 'absoloute safety'. In older patients the decision is not so obvious; very few patients have been found at operation to have locally involved resectable lymph nodes or residual tumor even when the histology appears 'unfavorable', but some patients found to have no residual cancer have died as a result of the (unnecessary) surgery. Operation does not, in any case, guarantee freedom from residual cancer; there have been reports of subsequent death from distant (micro-)metastases in spite of normal operative findings by the surgeon and histopathologist.

COMPLICATIONS

Bleeding is the most frequent complication of polypectomy, usually 'delayed' 1–14 days after polypectomy, but occasionally 'immediate' after transection. Bleeding (whether immediate or delayed) should complicate less than 1% of polypectomies. Hemorrhage from large polyp stalks has become rare as endoscopists have appreciated the need for maximum 'slow-cook' stalk electrocoagulation and the usefulness of epinephrine injection and nylon-loop or clip strangulation.

Immediate bleeding is usually a slow ooze but can be an arteriolar spurt of frightening proportions, as viewed endoscopically. Every possible attempt should be made to stop an arterial bleed immediately as any delay can result in the view being lost or in clot formation. Infusing large volumes of water prevents clotting if blood obscures the view of the bleeding point. Clots are impossible to aspirate but, with posturing to the right side if necessary to visualize the distal colon, localization of the polypectomy site and endoscopic therapy should be possible. Quickly re-snare the remaining stalk or inject epinephrine (up to 5–10 mL of 1 : 10 000 solution) submucosally into or adjacent to the stalk remnant. If the stalk has been re-snared, simple strangulation alone (taping the snare handle closed for 10–15 min) is usually sufficient without further electrocoagulation. If bleeding recurs on releasing the snare, attempts to stop it can be made with further electrocoagulation or by injection, if necessary using a second instrument (pediatric colonoscope or gastroscope) passed up alongside the first. In the unlikely event that arterial bleeding persists in spite of all efforts, the most elegant solution is to perform selective arterial catheterization and embolization or infusion of Pitressin® (success has been reported using Pitressin® or somatostatin by intravenous infusion alone). A surgical team must be alerted and adequate supplies of blood ensured.

Secondary (delayed) hemorrhage can occur for up to 12–14 days— particularly after snaring of larger polyps or hot biopsy of over-large (over 5 mm) polyps. Delayed bleeds may perhaps be more frequent or more persistent in patients on aspirin, which ideally should be stopped 7–10 days beforehand if multiple or large polypectomies are predicted. Persistent or secondary hemorrhage in the left colon will be indicated by repeated calls to stool and the passage of fresh clots, whereas in the right colon the rate of bleeding is more difficult to assess because of the long delay before altered blood is expelled.

All patients who have had polypectomy should know of the possibility of delayed bleeding, partly for reassurance sake if minor bleeding occurs, but also to be aware of the possible need to report to hospital for observation should blood loss be persistent or substantial. Hemorrhage from the distal colon will be indicated by repeated calls to stool and the passage of fresh clots, whereas in the proximal colon bleeding is more difficult to assess because of the long delay before altered blood is expelled. Delayed hemorrhage normally stops spontaneously but transfusion (and perhaps repeat colonoscopy) is occasionally required.

The 'post-polypectomy syndrome', with fever, pain and peritonism, represents 'closed perforation' with full-thickness heat damage to the bowel wall. It is an occasional sequel to a difficult polypectomy, especially after piecemeal removal of a large sessile polyp in the proximal colon. Localized abdominal pain and fever persist for 12–24 hours following polypectomy, but without free gas on X-ray or signs of generalized peritonitis. The inflammatory reaction of the peritoneum should result in adherence by local structures (typically covering by omentum or small bowel), so it is a self-limiting event. Conservative management with bed rest and systemic antibiotics is indicated, but surgical consultation is wise if the symptoms and signs do not abate rapidly.

Frank perforation is fortunately rare. Management may often be conservative, but this depends on the area of the polyp base. A small polyp removed by snare or hot biopsy in a well-prepared bowel is obviously 'low risk', whereas signs of perforation after a larger or sessile lesion in a poorly prepared colon mandate surgery. A surgeon should always be alerted; if in doubt, it is safest to operate.

SAFETY

Any polypectomy is potentially hazardous, so adherence to all possible safety measures is essential. Assuming that the correct equipment is available, it must be carefully handled and maintained. Never bend or coil the connecting leads tightly or they will fracture; if a lead looks or feels partially fractured, replace it or have it mended at once. If polypectomy is not proceeding according to plan, check the electrosurgical settings, connections and patient plate circuitry before anything else.

The greatest single safety factor lies in a strict routine, regularly repeated for each polypectomy, because human error is much more likely than equipment failure. A military-type approach has much to commend it: any request from the endoscopist being repeated out loud by the assistant so that each knows what the other is doing. The assistant and the endoscopist must check on each other to watch that all is in order during the procedure, having checked the equipment (including marking the snare handle at the point of closure) beforehand.

Good bowel preparation is essential to give a good view and a dry field in which to work. If bowel preparation is poor, as during flexible sigmoidoscopy, use carbon dioxide instead of air to prevent the possibility of explosive combinations of oxygen (from inflated air) with methane (from bacterial metabolism of protein residues) or hydrogen (from bacterial fermentation of carbohydrates). Alternatively, take great care to insufflate and then aspirate repeatedly to dilute any gas present. In a well-prepared bowel there is no explosion hazard and air can be safely used (see the caveat on mannitol bowel preparation, p. 94).

The endoscopist should be aware of the patient's *medications*. To minimize the risk of delayed hemorrhage, patient medication with aspirin, NSAIDs and other medications affecting platelet adhesion should ideally be withdrawn a week before (to allow a new generation of 'sticky' platelets to form), and for 7–14 days after the procedure. In practice most endoscopists will proceed with polypectomy even if the patient is found to be on antiplatelet medication, but with scrupulous attention to careful technique and due warning to the patient about the possibility of delayed bleeding.

Only a very experienced operator should undertake polypectomy in a patient on anticoagulants. The patient should be warned of the possible need for immediate repeat endoscopy should delayed bleeding occur, since spontaneous cessation is less likely. Very careful precautions should be taken for effective coagulation during polypectomy, and safety loops or clips perhaps placed afterwards. Often, with the approval of the relevant clinician, anticoagulants can be stopped for the 10–12-day period needed to cover the procedure and the likelihood of immediate or delayed bleeding after polypectomy. Some favor admission of the patient to hospital and transfer to heparin for the immediate postpolypectomy period, but the major risk of (delayed) bleeding comes later, often after discharge from hospital.

POLYPECTOMY OUTSIDE THE COLON

The principles described above are also applicable for gastric or duodenal polypectomy or for the resection of dysplastic or early malignant areas in the esophagus or stomach. Esophageal or gastric resections tend to be extensive and there is a higher risk of both bleeding and perforation when snaring duodenal polyps, compared with those in the colon. Snare-loop biopsy for diagnostic purposes (Ménétrier's disease, etc.) is useful in the stomach but some caution is needed because it is easy to take a much bigger bite than intended when assessing using a wide-angle of view in a large viscus. Gastric polyps are more often trivial and non-neoplastic than adenomatous, and tend to be small and easily managed; the innumerable shiny 'fundic gland polyps' in the gastric body and fundus of many FAP patients (and a few others) can be entirely ignored. Peutz–Jeghers polyps may be larger but are usually thin-stalked and easy to snare. It is wise to suppress gastric acid for 1 week after any upper GI polypectomy to reduce the likelihood of delayed hemorrhage. Gastric and duodenal resection specimens are easily lost after snaring, so use of antispasmodics and a quick eye and hand are desirable. A nylon retrieval net is the ideal means for safe retrieval of larger or multiple specimens because of the obvious need to safeguard the airways during withdrawal.

Perforation is more likely in the duodenum and small intestine because the wall is thin, so there is a corresponding need for greater caution in snaring and electrosurgery. The endoscopist's role in FAP patient upper GI tract surveillance is fortunately mainly limited to inspection at 1–3-yearly intervals, with representative biopsies for dysplasia grade. Papillary resection for high-grade dysplasia is a rare possibility. The large sessile polyps that occur in the peripapillary area of less than 10% of FAP patients are distinctly hazardous to remove except by endoscopic mucosal resection (EMR), whereas the frequent tiny polyps or pale dysplastic areas can be ignored. Polyps with severe dysplasia histologically or size approaching 1 cm require removal by mucosectomy or snaring. Open surgery, usually Whipple's operation (with subtotal pancreatectomy), is the 'last-ditch' option the endoscopist is seeking to avoid.

The technique of suction cap EMR has particular application for duodenal polypectomy as well as, more frequently, for 'piecemeal' removal of areas of high-grade dysplasia or early cancer in esophageal or gastric mucosa. It is rarely needed in the colon, since simple injection polypectomy is easier. Suction cap EMR requires a little endoscopic dexterity but is remarkably safe and effective:

1 Preload the transparent EMR suction cap onto the tip of the gastroscope (Fig. 7.43a).

2 If several resections are expected, also preload an overtube over the endoscope shaft.

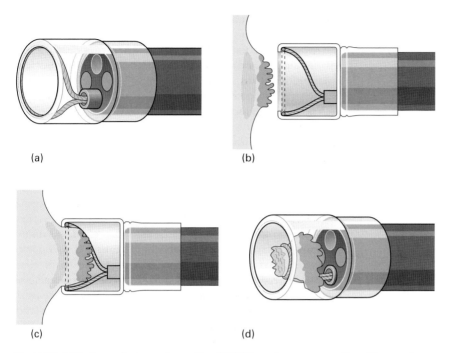

Fig. 7.43 (a) Endoscopic mucosal resection (EMR) lipped cap on scope tip, with snare loop opened. (b) Polyp elevated by injection. (c) Injected tissue suctioned in. (d) Electrosurgical snaring and transection.

3 Inject saline beneath the polyp or area of mucosa to be resected, to elevate it away from the muscular layer below and make excision safer and easier.

4 Suction the mucosa against the cap to help open the special EMR snare loop against the internal lip of the suction cap (unless this has been pre-loaded) (Fig. 7.43b).

5 Suction until the mucosa completely fills the transparent cap, becoming encircled by the EMR snare loop (Fig. 7.43c).

6 Snare off the specimen and suction it into the cap for withdrawal with the endoscope (Fig. 7.43d).

7 Reinsert the scope through the overtube for multiple resections—which can remove extensive areas of mucosa, if indicated.

OTHER THERAPEUTIC PROCEDURES

Balloon dilation

Balloon dilation of short strictures and anastomoses is easy with 'through-the-scope' (TTS) balloons, especially those with an internal guide wire. TTS balloons now furl tightly enough to pass through small-diameter instruments (although a standard 3.7 mm channel gives better feel and control). The balloon is silicone-spray lubricated before insertion. The instrument shaft and tip is straightened as much as practicable to minimize insertion force and avoid kinking (to achieve this it may be necessary to withdraw the scope a little and pass back to the stricture once the balloon is in position). The integral guide wire makes insertion through angulated or fixed strictured areas substantially easier, but considerable dexterity, handling skill and imagination are often needed to coax the balloon into position.

Balloons of at least 18 mm diameter give the best long-term results and those that are 5 cm long are easiest to 'dumb-bell' within the stricture, staying put rather than slipping in or out during distension. Balloons must be fluid-distended, using either water or dilute contrast material, because air is too compressible. A pressure-gun and manometer are used, because it is impossible by hand to reach and sustain the recommended distension pressures—typically around 5 bar or 80 psi (pounds per square inch)—for the 2 minutes needed to dilate effectively, especially as the balloon plastic slowly stretches a little. The gun also allows the pressure control needed for 'controlled radial expansion' balloons, which give the endoscopist a reasonably precise idea of the dilation diameter achieved.

Dilation is hazardous and how far to dilate is a matter of judgment. The overall perforation rate for stricture dilation in different series ranges between 5 and 10%, so seriously informed consent must be obtained beforehand, and the patient should appreciate that there is a small but significant risk of ending up in the operating theatre. Very scarred, ulcerated or angulated strictures are more likely to split under dilation (perhaps dilate to 12–15 mm initially and repeat to a larger diameter on another occasion). Postsurgical anastomotic strictures are safer and easier, especially if 'straight-on'. Metallic stents (see below) may have a place in managing the most obstinate and fibrous stenoses. On the other hand, the typically web-like fibrous bands that can occur at some anastomotic strictures are susceptible to 'needle-knife' incision before large-diameter balloon dilation, with excellent results.

Tube placement

Deflation and tube placement is important in ileus or 'pseudo-obstruction' (Ogilvie's syndrome), where endoscopic deflation avoids the need for surgery. Unless a drainage tube is left, ideally inserted into the proximal colon, simple colonic deflation tends to be short-lived in effect. Different methods are available.

A purpose-designed colon drainage set is available for 'through-the-scope' insertion, or components of an ERCP stent set can be used, cutting holes in the pusher tube before inserting it over the guide wire, leaving the tube behind and withdrawing the guide wire. Frequent irrigation of the tube is likely to be needed because of its small diameter.

A *'piggy-back' method carries up a larger drainage tube* alongside the scope, a loop attached to the leading end of the tube being grasped by forceps (Fig. 7.44). A variation avoids using the forceps and allows better suction during the procedure (the colon may be unprepared and foul); a thin loop of cotton thread at the end of the tube is held by a loop of strong monofilament nylon passed through the suction channel; once in the proximal colon a sharp tug on the nylon loop breaks the cotton thread and the tube is free. The drainage tube is attached to a suction pump or drainage bag. The tendency of the deflation tube to be ejected by colonic movement can be prevented by stiffening it with a guide wire (Savary–Guillard or similar steel-wire type), silicone-lubricated for insertion.

Volvulus and intussusception

The colonoscope can be used to deflate a *sigmoid volvulus*, effectively acting as a steerable flatus tube, so that the deflated loop can de-rotate passively. Large-channel colonoscopes allow a deflation tube (as above) to be inserted through the instrumentation channel. After the tube or endoscope tip is passed gently into or through the twisted segment, deflation alone is usually sufficient for the torsion to reverse spontaneously and endoscopic manipulation is usually unnecessary. However, if the segment appears blue-black and gangrenous from ischemia, surgery is indicated because of the high risk of perforation.

Intussusception is easy to diagnose but usually impossible to reduce colonoscopically, because not enough inward push can be transmitted around the looped colon to the ileo-cecal area (where this rare event most commonly occurs). Identifying and removing any causative factor, such as a large polyp or lipoma, should help prevent recurrence.

Angiodysplasia and hemangiomas

In treating angiodysplasia it is best to err on the side of applying too little heat. Even minor whitening and edema will progress to produce remarkable local ulceration within 24 hours. It is easy enough to repeat the examination a few weeks later to check results, but difficult to justify perforation from overaggression during the first procedure. Since angiodysplasias occur mainly in the thin-walled proximal colon, great care should be taken with whichever modality is used—preferably APC (argon plasma coagulation) for its ease, efficacy and relative safety; but, if this is unavailable, any other form of electrocoagulation (mono- or bipolar), heater probe or laser, can be carefully applied. The

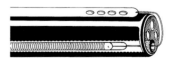

Fig. 7.44 A deflation tube can be carried up alongside the colonoscope.

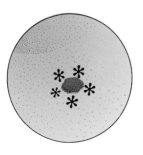

Fig. 7.45 Point coagulation around angiodysplasia before heating the center.

judicious use of hot biopsy forceps is particularly effective with smaller lesions, which can be grasped, the mucosa tented up and selectively heated. It is unnecessary to take a biopsy, and the jaws are simply reopened after minimal visible coagulation. In those larger angiodysplasias that have an obvious central 'feeding vessel' it is preferable to create a ring of local heating points around the periphery, followed by one or more applications near the center, rather than to apply excessive heat in one area alone and risk bleeding or perforation (Fig. 7.45).

Larger angiodysplasias should be tackled last, and the most dependent ones treated first, because they may bleed and cause others to be missed. The object of coagulation is to damage the superficial part of the vascular lesion (which extends also into the submucosa) coagulating the vessels nearest the surface that are most liable to trauma, but also causing regrowth of normal mucosa over the top of the remaining vessels. If several angiodysplasias are present it can be difficult to be certain which has been the source of bleeding. Surface ulceration is a rare but obvious pointer; a small bright-red lesion, well perfused from below, is more suspect than a larger but superficial, spidery and pinkish one. Mucosal trauma or spots of blood are easy to mistake for angiodysplasia; if in doubt irrigate the surface or traumatize the 'lesion' to see if it bleeds—better than overdiagnosing and risking a complication unnecessarily.

Hemangiomas invariably have snake-like, very tortuous, vessels. There is great variation in colon vessel pattern, and a corresponding tendency to overdiagnose vascular abnormality. Endoscopic therapy is in any case ineffective in generalized hemangiomas; simply document the appearance. Only the rare polypoid protuberances of childhood 'cavernous hemangiomas' (blue rubber bleb nevus syndrome) are endoscopically treatable, whether by APC or sclerotherapy (they can occur throughout the GI tract, as well as in the skin and elsewhere).

Tumor destruction and palliation

Debulking and vaporization of inoperable or obstructing tumor tissue is possible, using any combination of snaring, APC or laser photocoagulation. Multiple injections of 100% ethanol using a sclerotherapy needle have also been used, the procedure being repeated every day or two until the desired clearance is achieved. In the rectum a urological resectoscope loop has been used, as for transurethral prostatectomy, either under glycine solution or in air.

Insertion of self-expanding metal stents has largely replaced such heroics. The stents used are similar to esophageal stents but, partly because tumor in-growth is slow and easily managed but stent migration a problem, colonic stents are uncoated and their Nitonol 'memory metal' construction deliberately made to be immovable (so also unremovable). Insertion of colonic stents is normally a combined endoscopic-fluoroscopic procedure. Ideally the endoscopist inserts the scope proximal to the tumor, passing the guide wire and allowing precise localization of the upper and lower margins either by means of metal clips or radiological skin markers. Occasionally formal dilation may be needed, but usually there is slow spontaneous (and much safer) dilation of the stent over the next 24 hours. If an endoscope will not pass the strictured area a hydrophilic 'J-wire' can be inserted under direct vision, contrast injected down its catheter and the rest of the procedure and stent insertion managed under fluoroscopic control. The endoscopist checks for satisfactory location and expansion of the distal end of the stent.

FURTHER READING

Polypectomy techniques

Barlow, DE. Endoscopic applications of electrosurgery: a review of basic principles. *Gastrointest Endosc* 1982; 28: 73–6.

Binmoeller KF, Bohnacker S, Seifert H, Thonke F, Valdeyar H, Soehendra N. Endoscopic snare excision of "giant" colorectal polyps. *Gastrointest Endosc* 1996; 43: 183–8.

Canard JM, Vedrenne B. Clinical application of argon plasma coagulation in gastrointestinal endoscopy: has the time come to replace the laser? *Endoscopy* 2001; 33: 353–7.

Grund KE, Straub T, Farin G. New haemostatic techniques: argon plasma coagulation. *Best Pract Res Clin Gastroenterol* 1999; 13: 67–84.

Tappero G, Gaia E, DeGiuli P *et al.* Cold snare excision of small colorectal polyps. *Gastrointest Endosc* 1992; 38: 310–13.

Wadas DD, Sanowski RA. Complications of the hot-biopsy forceps technique. *Gastrointest Endosc* 1987; 33: 32–7.

Waye JD. New methods of polypectomy. *Gastrointest Endosc Clin North Am* 1997; 7: 413–22.

Clinical aspects of polypectomy

Brooker JC, Saunders BP, Shah SG, Thapar CJ, Suzuki N, Williams CB. Treatment with argon plasma coagulation reduces recurrence after piecemeal resection of large sessile colonic polyps: a randomized trial and recommendations. *Gastrointest Endosc* 2002; 55: 371–5.

Cappell MS, Abdullah M. Management of gastrointestinal bleeding induced by gastrointestinal endoscopy. *Gastroenterol Clin North Am* 2000; 29: 125–7.

Clements RH, Jordan LM, Webb WA. Critical decisions in the management of endoscopic perforations of the colon. *Am Surg* 2000; 66: 91–3.

Cranley JP, Petras RE, Carey WD, Paradis K, Sivak MV. When is endoscopic polypectomy adequate therapy for colonic polyps containing invasive carcinoma? *Gastroenterology* 1986; 91: 419–27.

Ellis KK, Fennerty MB. Marking and identifying colon lesions. Tattoos, clips, and radiology in imaging the colon. *Gastrointest Endosc Clin North Am* 1997; 7: 401–11.

Giardiello FM, Welsh SB, Hamilton SR *et al.* Peutz–Jeghers syndrome: perhaps not so benign. *N Engl J Med* 1987; 316: 1511–14.

Haggitt RC, Glotzbach RE, Soffer EE, Wruble LD. Prognostic factors in colorectal carcinomas arising in adenomas: implications for lesions removed by endoscopic polypectomy. *Gastroenterology* 1985; 89: 328–36.

Hoff G. Colorectal polyps. Clinical implications: screening and cancer prevention. *Scand J Gastroenterol* 1987; 22: 769–75.

Hofstad B, Vatn MH, Andersen SN, Huitfeldt HS, Rognum T, Larsen S, Osnes M. Growth of colorectal polyps: redetection and evaluation of unresected polyps for a period of three years. *Gut* 1996; 39: 449–56.

Hofstad B, Vatn M. Growth rate of colon polyps and cancer. [Review]. *Gastrointest Endosc Clin North Am* 1997; 7: 345–63.

Jass JR. Do all colorectal carcinomas arise in pre-existing adenomas? *World J Surg* 1989; 13: 45–51.

Ransohoff DF, Lang CA, Kuo HS. Colonoscopic surveillance after polypectomy: considerations of cost effectiveness. *Ann Int Med* 1991; 114: 177–81.

Rex DK, Lehman GA, Hawes RH, Ulbright TM, Smith JJ. Screening colonoscopy in asymptomatic average-risk persons with negative fecal occult blood tests. *Gastroenterology* 1991; 100: 64–7.

Waye JD. Endoscopic mucosal resection of colon polyps. *Gastrointest Endosc Clin North Am* 2001; 11: 537–48.

Williams CB, Saunders PB. The rationale for current practice in the management of malignant colonic polyps. *Endoscopy* 1993; 25: 469–74.

Winawer SJ, Zauber AG, May Nah Ho MS *et al.* Prevention of colorectal cancer by colonoscopic polypectomy. *N Engl J Med* 1993; 329: 1977–81.

Winawer SJ, Zauber AG, O'Brien MJ, May Nah Ho MS, Gottlieb L. Randomised comparison of surveillance intervals after colonoscopic removal of newly diagnosed adenomatous polyps. *N Engl J Med* 1993; 328: 901–6.

Zlatanic J, Waye JD, Kim PS, Baiocco PJ, Gleim GW. Large sessile colonic adenomas: use of argon plasma coagulator to supplement piecemeal snare polypectomy. *Gastrointest Endosc* 1999; 49: 731–5.

Stenting

Khot W, Lang AW, Murali K, Parker MC. Systematic review of the efficacy and safety of colorectal stents. *Br J Surg* 2002; 89(9): 1096–102.

Resources and Links

PROFESSIONAL SOCIETIES

American Gastroenterological Association (AGA)
7910 Woodmont Avenue Suite 700
Bethesda, MD 20814 USA
www.gastro.com

American College of Gastroenterology (ACG)
4900 B South 31st Street
Arlington, VA 22206-1656 USA
www.acg.gi.org

American Society for Gastrointestinal Endoscopy (ASGE)
13 Elm Street
Manchester, MA 01944 USA
www.asge.org

British Society of Gastroenterology (BSG)
3 St. Andrews Place
Regent's Park
London NW1 4LB, England
www.bsg.org.uk

ENDOSCOPY BOOKS

Annuals of Gastrointestinal Endoscopy, Cotton PB, Williams CB, Tytgat
   GNJ. Current Science, 1988–1998.
Annual reviews of the 'state of the art' in different endoscopy topics by
   international experts.

Classen M, Lightdale CJ, Tytgat GNJ. *Gastroenterological Endoscopy*.
   Thieme Stuttgart, New York, 2002: 777 pp.
A comprehensive multi-author review.

Cotton PB, Williams CB. *Practical Gastrointestinal Endoscopy* (4th edn).
   Oxford: Blackwell Science 1996.

DiMarino AJ, Benjamin SB. *Gastrointestinal Disease and Endoscopic Approach*. Boston: Blackwell Science Inc, 1997.
A comprehensive two volume textbook (1161 pages), focusing on the
   clinical practice of gastrointestinal endoscopy.

Gastrointestinal Endoscopy Clinics of North America (series ed. Sivak MV).

Fox VL. *Pediatric gastrointestinal endoscopy. Gastrointestinal Endoscopy Clinics of North America*, Vol. 11(4) (series ed. Sivak MV), Philadelphia: WB Saunders, 2001.

Gostout C, ed. *Treatment of variceal bleeding. Gastrointestinal Endoscopy Clinics of North America*, Vol. 9(2) (series ed. Lightdale CJ), Philadelphia: WB Saunders, 1999.

Kozarek RA. *Endoscopic disinfection and reprocessing of endoscopic accessories. Gastrointestinal Endoscopy Clinics of North America*, Vol. 10(2) (series ed. Sivak MV), Philadelphia: WB Saunders, 2000.

Leung JW, Lee JG, eds. *Nonvariceal upper gastrointestinal bleeding. Gastrointestinal Endoscopy Clinics of North America*, Vol. 7(4) (series ed. Sivak MV), Philadelphia: WB Saunders, 1997.

Marcon NE, ed. *Management of esophageal stenosis. Gastrointestinal Endoscopy Clinics of North America*, Vol. 8(2) (series ed. Sivak MV), Philadelphia: WB Saunders, 1998.

Shike M, Bloch AS, eds. *Enteral nutrition. Gastrointestinal Endoscopy Clinics of North America*, Vol. 8(3) (series ed. Sivak MV), Philadelphia: WB Saunders, 1998.

Weinstein WM, ed. *Endoscopic biopsy. Gastrointestinal Endoscopy Clinics of North America*, Vol. 10(4) (series ed. Sivak MV), Philadelphia: WB Saunders, 2000.

Greene FL, Ponsky JL. *Endoscopic Surgery*. Philadelphia: WB Saunders, 1994.

Modlin IM. *A Brief History of Endoscopy*. Milano: Multimed, 2000.
Not so brief—a fascinating and detailed historical review, including the history of endoscopic societies.

Schiller KFR, Cockel R, Hunt RH, Warren BF. *Atlas of Gastrointestinal Endoscopy and Related Pathology* (2nd edn). Oxford: Blackwell Science, 2002.
Detailed text and multiple images, incorporating pathology.

Shepherd M, Mason J, Swan CJ. *Practical Endoscopy*. Chapman Hall Medical, 1997.
An excellent introduction aimed primarily at nurses and endoscopy assistants.

Sivak M (ed.). *Gastroenterologic Endoscopy* (2nd edn). Philadelphia: WB
    Saunders, 2000.
The biggest textbook to date (120 contributing authors, 1611 pages).

Steele RJC, Chung SCS, Leung JWC. *Practical Management of Acute Gas-
    trointestinal Bleeding.* Oxford: Butterworth-Heinemann, 1993.

ENDOSCOPY JOURNALS

Gastrointestinal Endoscopy
The official journal of the ASGE.
Publishers: Mosby
Editor: Michael V. Sivak.
University Hospitals of Cleveland (Wearn 253)
11100 Euclid Avenue
Cleveland, OH 44106-5066

Endoscopy
Official journal of the European Society of Gastrointestinal
Endoscopy (ESG), and 20 affiliated national societies. Editor-in-
Chief M. Classen
Publishers: Georg Thieme Verlag
Postfach 30 11 20
70451 Stuttgart, Germany
http://www.thieme.connect.com

Surgical Endoscopy
Official journal of the Society of American Gastrointestinal
Endoscopic Surgeons (SAGES) and European Association for
Endoscopic surgery (EAES)
Publishers: Springer-Verlag New York Inc.
Bruce V. MacFadyen, Jr, Sir Alfred Cuschieri,Editors-in-Chief
http.//link.springer.de/link/service/journals

Digestive Endoscopy
Official Journal of the Japan Gastroenterological Endoscopy
Society
Publishers: Blackwell Publishing Ltd.
http://www.blackwellpublishing.com

WEBSITES

American College of Gastroenterology, http://www.acg.gi.org
American   Gastroenterological   Association,   http://
www.gastro.com
American Society for Gastrointestinal Endoscopy, http://
www.asge.org
British Society of Gastroenterology, http://www.bsg.org.uk
MUSC Digestive Disease Center, http://www.ddc.musc.edu

GastroHep, http://www.gastroHep.com–a resource for practising gastroenterologists, endoscopists and hepatologists

GUIDELINES FOR ENDOSCOPY

http://www.gastrohep.com/guidelines (a comprehensive and searchable collection from all sources)

ASGE Guidelines—Privileging and credentialing

Endoscopy by non-physicians skills. *Gastrointest Endosc* 1999; 49: 826–8.

Guidelines for credentialing and granting privileges for gastrointestinal endoscopy. *Gastrointest Endosc* 2002; 55: 780–3.

Methods of privileging for new technology in gastrointestinal endoscopy. *Gastrointest Endosc* 1999; 50: 899–900.

Proctoring and hospital endoscopy privileges. *Gastrointest Endosc* 1999; 50: 901–5.

Renewal of endoscopic privileges. *Gastrointest Endosc* 1999; 49: 823–5.

ASGE Guidelines–Training

Guidelines for training in patient monitoring and sedation and analgesia. *Gastrointest Endosc* 1998; 49: 669–71.

Principles of training in gastrointestinal endoscopy. *Gastrointest Endosc* 1999; 49: 845–53.

British Society of Gastroenterology Clinical Practice Guidelines (www.bsg.org.uk/clinical_prac/guidelines.htm)

Provision of endoscopy-related services in district general hospitals, 2001.

Antibiotic prophylaxis in gastrointestinal endoscopy, 2001.

Informed consent for endoscopic procedures, 1999.

Cleaning and disinfection of equipment for gastrointestinal endoscopy, 1997.

Index